NEW ASPECTS IN MOLECULAR AND CELLULAR MECHANISMS OF HUMAN CARCINOGENESIS

Edited by **Dmitry Bulgin**

New Aspects in Molecular and Cellular Mechanisms of Human Carcinogenesis
http://dx.doi.org/10.5772/59826
Edited by Dmitry Bulgin

Contributors
Mohamed Farouk El-Refaei, Anca Botezatu, Julio Cesar Osorio, Andres Castillo, Satoru Matsuda, Reigh-Yi Lin, Dmitry Bulgin

Published by InTech
Janeza Trdine 9, 51000 Rijeka, Croatia

Publishing Process Manager Iva Lipovic
Technical Editor InTech DTP team
Cover InTech Design team

First published February, 2016
Printed in Croatia

Additional hard copies can be obtained from orders@intechopen.com

New Aspects in Molecular and Cellular Mechanisms of Human Carcinogenesis, Edited by Dmitry Bulgin
p. cm.
ISBN 978-953-51-2253-1

For EU product safety concerns:
IN TECH d.o.o., Prolaz Marije Krucifikse Kozulić 3, 51000 Rijeka, Croatia,
info@intechopen.com or visit our website at intechopen.com.

Meet the editor

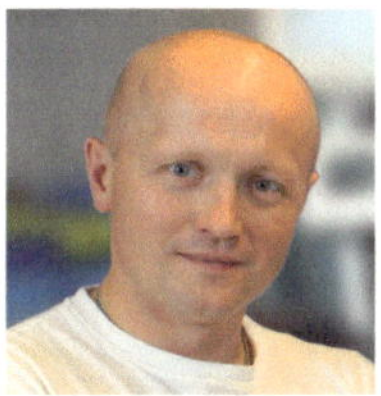

Dmitry Bulgin received his MD and PhD degrees from Smolensk State Medical University in 1998 and 2004, respectively. He served as an Assistant Professor at the Department of Pathology in Smolensk State Medical University from 2000 to 2004. Between 2004 and 2006, he has been a visiting researcher at the Department of Molecular Medicine of Atomic Bomb Disease Institute in Nagasaki University Graduate School of Biomedical Sciences. Since 2006, he was appointed as a Chairman of the Department of Laboratory Medicine at Pokrovskaya Municipal Hospital in Saint Petersburg, Russia. From 2010, he served as a principal research scientist and general practitioner at the Center for Regenerative Medicine ME-DENT in Rovinj, Croatia.
He is a member of professional associations such as Croatian Medical Chamber, European Society of Pathology, European Society for Artificial Organs, The Transplantation Society, European Radiation Research Society, and Tissue Engineering and Regenerative Medicine International Society. His research interests include Cancer Research, Stem Cell Biology, Molecular Medicine, Ionizing Radiation, and Tissue Regeneration.

Contents

Preface

Intensive research efforts during the past several decades have increased our understanding of carcinogenesis and have identified a cellular and molecular basis for the multi-step process of cancer development. Technological advances in molecular biology have proven invaluable to the understanding of the pathogenesis of human cancer. The application of molecular techniques to the study of cancer has not only led to advances in tumor diagnosis and development of new treatment approaches but also provided markers for the assessment of prognosis and disease progression.

I wish to thank all the authors of this book for their excellent contributions. They share my hope that this book provides an update on recent progress in some key areas of cancer research and assists other scientists in the better understanding of the molecular pathogenesis of cancer.

I would like to express my gratitude my mentor, professor Shunichi Yamashita (Nagasaki University, Japan), and to my colleague, professor Serik Meirmanov (Ritsumeikan Asia Pacific University, Japan) for their professional support in the fields of cancer research and radiation biology.

Dmitry Bulgin
Center for Regenerative Medicine "ME-DENT",
Rovinj
Croatia

Chapter 1

Mechanisms of Oncogene Activation

Anca Botezatu, Iulia V. Iancu, Oana Popa, Adriana Plesa, Dana Manda, Irina Huica, Suzana Vladoiu, Gabriela Anton and Corin Badiu

Additional information is available at the end of the chapter

http://dx.doi.org/10.5772/61249

Abstract

The main modifications that characterize cancer are represented by alterations in oncogenes, tumor-suppressor genes, and non-coding RNA genes. Most of these alterations are somatic and the process is a multistep one. Tumors often arise from an initial transformed cell, and after subsequent genetic alterations different cytogenetically clones lead to tumor heterogeneity.

Oncogenes encode proteins that control cell processes such as proliferation and apoptosis. Among these proteins are transcription factors, chromatin remodelers, growth factors, growth factor receptors, signal transducers, and apoptosis regulators. Oncogenes activation by structural alteration (chromosomal rearrangement, gene fusion, mutation, and gene amplification) or epigenetic modification (gene promoter hypomethylation, microRNA expression pattern) confers an increased or a deregulated expression. Therefore, cells with such alterations possess a growth advantage or an increased survival rate. Given the fact that expression profiling of these alterations determines specific signatures associated with tumor classification, diagnosis, staging, prognosis, and response to treatment, it highlights the importance of studying oncogenes activation mechanisms and the great potential that they hold as therapeutic tools in the near future.

Keywords: Oncogenes, genomic instability, epigenetic modification

1. Introduction

The main modifications that characterize cancer are represented by alterations in oncogenes, tumor-suppressor genes, and non-coding RNA genes. Most of these alterations are somatic and the process is a multistep one, although germ-line mutations can predispose a person to heritable or familial cancer.

Tumors often arise from an initial transformed cell, and after subsequent genetic alterations different cytogenetically clones lead to tumor heterogeneity. Tumor heterogeneity determines different clinical phenotypes, leading to an individual response to treatment for tumors with the same diagnostic type.

Oncogenes encode proteins that control cell processes such as proliferation and apoptosis. Among these proteins are transcription factors, chromatin remodelers, growth factors, growth factor receptors, signal transducers, and apoptosis regulators. Activation of oncogenes by structural alterations (chromosomal rearrangement, gene fusion, mutation, and gene amplification) or epigenetic modification (gene promoter hypomethylation) confers an increased or a deregulated expression. Therefore, cells with such alterations possess a growth advantage or an increased survival rate. Translocations and mutations occur early on in tumor progression, whereas amplification usually occurs during late tumor stages.

A proto-oncogene is a normal gene that presents a potential to become an oncogene after a genetic alteration (mutation), leading to an increased expression. Usually, proto-oncogenes code for proteins that control cell growth and differentiation through signal transduction and execution of mitogenic signals. Upon activation, a proto-oncogene (or its product onco-protein) becomes a tumor-inducing agent. Most known examples of proto-oncogenes include *RAS, WNT, MYC, ERK*, and *TRK*. Another oncogene is the *BCR-ABL* gene found on the Philadelphia chromosome, a piece of genetic material seen in chronic myelogenous leukemia caused by the translocation of pieces from chromosomes 9 and 22 t (9; 22).

Oncogene products can comprise a variety of molecules such as transcription factors, chromatin remodelers, growth factors, growth factor receptors, signal transducers, and apoptosis regulators, each playing an important role in neoplastic transformation. For example, studies have shown that in prostate carcinomas the fusion between the *TMPR552* gene and two transcription factors *ERG*1 or *ETV1* creates a fusion protein that increases proliferation and inhibits apoptosis of cells in the prostate gland, thereby facilitating their transformation into cancer cells [1]. Another example is represented by chromatin remodeler factors such as the *MLL* gene that plays a critical role in acute lymphocytic leukemia and acute myelogenous leukemia [2]. Also, an essential role in cancer development is played by apoptosis regulators such as the *BCL2* gene, which is involved in the initiation of almost all follicular lymphomas and some diffuse large B-cell lymphomas [3].

2. Mutations

Mutations in an oncogene may lead to a change in the structure of encoded protein, enhancing its transforming activity. Oncogenes are activated by point mutations (substitutions) and may either enhance or degrade the function of a protein. Table 1 shows the occurrences of mutations in each oncogene among some tissues [4].

http://dx.doi.org/10.5772/61249

CANCER TYPE	ONCOGENES		TYPE
T cell lymphoma	*KIT*	*KRAS*	Co-occurred
Acute lymphoblastic leukemia	*KRAS*	*NRAS*	Co-occurred
Acute myeloid leukemia	*KRAS*	*NRAS*	Co-occurred
	FLT3	*KIT*	Mutually exclusive
Lung adenocarcinoma	*BRAF*	*KRAS*	Mutually exclusive
	KRAS	*NRAS*	Mutually exclusive
	EGFR3	*KRAS*	Mutually exclusive
Pancreatic cancer	*B-CATENIN*	*KRAS*	Mutually exclusive
Biliary tract cancer	*BRAF*	*KRAS*	Mutually exclusive
Colorectal cancer	*BRAF*	*KRAS*	Mutually exclusive
	KRAS	*PIK3CA*	Co-occurred
	B-CATENIN	*KRAS*	Co-occurred
	KRAS	*NRAS*	Mutually exclusive
Thyroid cancer	*BRAF*	*NRAS*	Mutually exclusive
	HRAS	*NRAS*	Mutually exclusive
	BRAF	*RET*	Mutually exclusive
	NRAS	*RET*	Mutually exclusive
Melanoma	*BRAF*	*NRAS*	Mutually exclusive
	BRAF	*HRAS*	Mutually exclusive
	BRAF	*KRAS*	Mutually exclusive
	KRAS	*BRAS*	Co-occurred
Prostate cancer	*HRAS*	*NRAS*	Mutually exclusive
	KRAS	*NRAS*	Mutually exclusive
Kidney cancer	*B-CATENIN*	*WTI*	Co-occurred
Cervical cancer	*PIK3CA*	*KRAS*	Mutually exclusive
	PIK3CA	*BRAF*	Mutually exclusive

Table 1. Frequently mutated oncogenes in various type of cancers

In cancer, mutations occur in many oncogenes, most notable being *RAS* and *BRAF*. The *RAS* family represents the upstream component of the RAS/RAF/MAPK pathway and mutations in *RAS* are one of the most common activating events in most of cancers. Mutated *RAS* oncogene (*KRAS, HRAS*, and *NRAS*) encodes for a protein that remains in the active state and transduces signals for continuous cell growth. *KRAS* mutations are common in carcinomas of the lung, colon, and pancreas [5], whereas mutations of *NRAS* occur in acute myelogenous leukemia and the myelodysplastic syndrome [6].

BRAF is a protein member of the *RAF* family (RAF1, BRAF, ARAF), also regulated by RAS binding. Mutated *BRAF* oncogene encodes for a protein with a modified kinase domain, resulting in a constitutively active protein that uncontrollably stimulates the MAP kinase cascade [7].

2.1. Melanoma

BRAF mutations are the most common somatic mutations in cutaneous melanoma and are extremely rare in mucosal melanoma. There are found in 48% of metastatic biopsy specimens and can precede neoplastic transformation [8, 9]. Over 90% of the identified mutations in *BRAF* are in codon 600. The most common is *BRAFV600E,* resulting in substitution of glutamic acid for valine (*BRAFV600E*: nucleotide 1799 T>A; codon GTG>GAG). The second most common mutation is *BRAFV600K* (5–6%) substituting lysine for valine, (GTG>AAG), followed by *BRAFV600R* (GTG>AGG), *BRAFV600′E2′* (GTG>GAA). Less common *BRAF* mutations found in cutaneous melanoma are *BRAF V600D* (GTG>GAT) and *L597R* [10–12].

There were identified mutations in hotspot codons (12, 13, and 61) of different *RAS* genes (*HRAS, NRAS,* or *KRAS*), but the most prevalent were *HRAS* substitutions that occurred preponderent at codon 61 (*HRAS Q61L* mutation), with fewer mutations at codon 12 and codon 13 [13]. Mutations in *N-RAS* appear to be significant in melanoma even earlier than the discovery of *BRAF* mutations [14]. The base change at position 61 seems to be important in the activation of *N-RAS* genes, transforming activity being detected only when mutant codon 61 was present. *BRAFV600E* mutations are more common in younger persons and in tumors arising from intermittently sun-exposed skin, exclusive with *N-RAS* [15].

C-KIT gene encodes a receptor tyrosine kinase (KIT). All the mutations were founded in exon 11, 13, and 17. The most common is V559A mutation that results in an amino acid substitution at position 559 in KIT, from a valine (V) to an alanine (A) [16]. While BRAF and NRAS mutations are common and significant in cutaneous melanomas, C-KIT mutations were detected in acral melanomas, mucosal melanomas, conjunctival melanomas, and cutaneous melanomas [17]

2.2. Colorectal cancer

The development of colorectal cancer (CRC) is a multistep process that occurs due to the accumulation of several genetic alterations, which are associated with oncogenes and tumor suppressor genes, as well as genes involved in DNA damage recognition and repair.

Most of the *BRAF* mutations associated with CRC are located in exons 11 and 15, coding for the kinase domain. The hotspot mutation at 1796 nucleotide is the T-to-A transversion that corresponds to the *V600E* mutation (7–15%) [18].

In colorectal cancer, *RAS* gene mutations have been reported in 40–50% and the frequency of *KRAS* mutations varies between 24–50%. *KRAS* mutation occurs most commonly in codon 12 and 13 rather than in codon 61, with the most frequent mutations: *G12D, G12V, G12C, G13D, Q61H* [19]. *KRAS* mutations exist in the presence of a vast majority of wild-type *KRAS* cells, which is why they not are detected in initial disease. Thirty-eight percent of patients whose tumors were initially *KRAS* wild-type developed *KRAS* mutations that were detectable in their sera after 5–6 months of treatment [20]. *KRAS* is mutated much more frequently than *NRAS*. *KRAS* mutations were studied to determine their role in the predictability of response to chemotherapy treatment.

2.3. Thyroid cancer

RAS mutations in thyroid cancer occur in both benign tumors and thyroid cancers (both papillary thyroid carcinoma (PTC) and follicular thyroid cancer (FTC)), with variable frequency in anaplastic thyroid cancers. PTCs with *RAS* mutations tend to display a lower rate of lymph node metastasis [21]. PTCs with *RAS* mutations often present a follicular architecture and a follicular variant of papillary thyroid carcinoma (FVPTC). There are two most common *RAS* mutations associated with thyroid cancer: mutations of *H-RAS* codon 61 and *N-RAS* codon 61 [22].

BRAF mutations were first detected missense mutations in thyroid cancer [23], which occurs in exon 15, due to the substitution of the amino acid valine for glutamic acid at residue position 600 [24]. This mutation is the most frequent genetic change in PTC [25], being found in 36–69% of PTC cases. *BRAF* mutation is responsible for the suppression of the sodium/iodide symporter (NIS), which is involved in iodine metabolism [26]. The *V600E* mutation comprises more than 90% of observed *BRAF* mutations, with the highest rate (77%) in the tall cell variant of papillary cancer, and the lowest percentage (12%) in the FVPTC. In PTC, *BRAF* mutation is more frequent in older patients, associated with extrathyroidal invasion [27]. By contrast, others have found that the *BRAF* mutation is not associated with age, gender, multicentricity, recurrence rate, lymphovascular invasion, or distant metastasis [28].

Activating point mutations of *RET* oncogenes are associated with hereditary cancer syndrome (multiple endocrine neoplasia type 2 -MEN 2). *RET* mutations are mostly missense and located in exons 10, 11 (extracellular domain of RET), 13, 14, 15, and 16 (in the TK domain) [29–31]. Mutation of the extracellular cysteine in codon 634 in exon 11 of RET causes ligand-independent dimerization of receptor molecules and enhances phosphorylation of intracellular substrates and cell transformation. Mutation of the intracellular TK (codon 918) results in cellular transformation [32].

There is a high correlation between the position of the point mutation and the phenotype of the disease. Three subtypes based on clinical presentation are defined: MEN 2A, MEN 2B, and FMTC. *RET* mutations are observed in 98% of MEN2A, 95% of MEN 2B, and 88% of familial medullary thyroid carcinoma (FMTC) [33]. Activating mutations of *RET* involving exons 10, 11, 13, 14, and 15 (encoding the highly conserved cysteine-rich domain) have been proven to cause MEN2A. [34]. The mutations for MEN2A are mostly located in exon 10 (10–15%), including codons 609, 611, 618, and 620, and exon 11 (80–85%), as well as codons 630 and 634 [35]. The mutations characteristic of FMTC occur in exons 10 and 11. However, non-cysteine point mutations also have been found in exon 8 (codons 532 and 533), exon 13 (codons 768, 790, and 791), exon 14 (codons 804 and 844), exon 15 (codon 891), and exon 16 (codon 912) [35–

37]. About 95% of MEN2B patients carry a *M918T* mutation within exon 16 and 5% have an *A883F* mutation in exon 15. Mutation in codon 918 gives a more aggressive phenotype [38].

2.4. Hepatocellular Carcinomas (HCC)

In HCC, only one mutation (*KRAS* codon 13; Gly to Asp) was detected among patients and no mutations were found in codons 12 and 61 of *KRAS* or codons 12, 13, and 61 of the *NRAS* and *HRAS* genes. So, the activation of *RAS* oncogenes by point mutations does not play a major role in hepatocellular carcinogenesis [39]. Activating mutations in the *BRAF* oncogene have been found in a small fraction of hepatocellular carcinomas. *KRAS* and *BRAF* mutations are rare events in HCC and therefore not a key event in hepatocarcinogenesis [40].

2.5. Pancreatic cancer

The highest incidence of *KRAS* mutations are found in adenocarcinomas of the pancreas (90%), with activating point mutations in codon 12 of the KRAS protein, leading to a glycine (G) to aspartic acid (D) or valine (V) substitution [41]. Single amino acid substitutions at G12, 13, or Q61 lead to the formation of mutated *KRAS* that are insensitive to GAP stimulation. This leads to the accumulation of persistently GTP-bound and active KRAS, which leads to pancreatic cancer formation [42].

2.6. Cervical cancer

Cervical cancer harbors high rates of potentially targetable oncogenic mutations. *KRAS* mutations were identified in low percentage (17%) exclusively in cervical adenocarcinomas. Most mutations were missense mutations of codon G12, well-described activating mutations, which have been associated with a worse prognosis in the metastatic process [43].

EGFR mutations were identified in 7.5% of cervical squamous cell carcinomas; a missense mutation in exon 15 of the *EGFR* gene produces an alternate spliced transcript (isoform D). Its presence in both tumor and adjacent normal tissue suggests that EGFR S703F may be a germline mutation [44, 45].

PIK3CA mutations are present in both squamous cell carcinomas and adenocarcinomas (31%). The *PIK3CA* mutations were located in the exon 9 helical domain in two hotspot mutations (*E545K* and *E542K*), which result in the constitutive activation of cellular signaling [46]. *PI3KCA* mutations may impart a more aggressive and treatment-resistant phenotype and decreased survival among patients with these mutations in early stage cancers [47].

3. Gene amplification and chromosomal translocations

The interest regarding the role of genomic context in promoting amplification was intensely investigated, but is still under debate. An important interest remains to establish the tendency of some genomic region to be subject to amplification. Past researches showed that different regions of the genome were more subjected to be amplified than others, but the molecular substrate was unknown [48]. At present, several mechanisms and models have been proposed to explain gene amplification in oncogenesis.

3.1. Gene amplification

Besides point mutations resulting in amino acid substitutions, a proto-oncogene may be activated by chromosomal alterations. Among the most important cromosomal abnormalities is gene amplification, which is an increase of the copy number for a specific chromosomal region. The consequence of chromosome fragment amplification is associated with overexpression of the amplified gene(s) and is a characteristic of cancer [49]. Amplified genes (hundreds of copies of normally diploid genes) may be organized as extrachromosomal elements (double minute chromosomes) as repeated units at a single locus or scattered throughout the genome.

At this moment, the relationships between the two forms of gene amplification found in tumors, the intrachromosomal homogeneously staining regions (HSRs) and the extrachromosomal DNA molecules, double minutes (dmins), are not well understood [50].

Several models for initiation of amplification have been described involving defects in DNA replication or telomere dysfunction and chromosomal fragile sites. Regarding the DNA replication initial proposals, based on extra rounds of replication due to replication origins misfiring appear to be incorrect modification of models invoking replication of extrachromosomal DNA [51]. Another theory involves the double-strand DNA breaks (frequent in replicating cells) generated by the collapse of replication forks that are unable to progress due to DNA structure lesions, therefore providing an opportunity to initiate the amplification process [49].

Telomeres are repetitive nucleotide sequences, with the role to prevent the loss of DNA sequences, resulted as a consequence of the incomplete DNA replication at the chromosome ends. Telomere shortening can block cell division; this mechanism appears to prevent genomic instability and development of cancer in aged cells by limiting the number of cell divisions [52]. Telomerase is responsible for telomere replication and is inactive in most somatic cells. With every cell division, the DNA telomere sequence is shortened by 40–50 bp. Telomere shortening in humans can induce replicative senescence, which blocks cell division. When telomeres are short to a critical length (replicative limit), cellular senescence is induced and normal cells cease to proliferate. This mechanism appears to prevent genomic instability and development of cancer in aged cells by limiting the number of cell divisions. In cancer, tumor cells escape replicative limit and acquire the capability to maintain telomere length through cell divisions by telomerase reactivation, or by using a recombination-based mechanism and alternate lengthening of telomeres (ALT) [53, 54]. An experimental murine model (lacking the RNA component of telomerase-TercK/K mice) for telomere dysfunction demonstrated the promotion of gene amplification. Tumor genomes arising in mutant mice contain chromosomal rearrangements, amplifications, and deletions commonly associated with human tumors [55, 56]. Despite the established correlation between telomerase reactivation and telomeres lengthening in cancer, recent literature review and analysis [52] suggest this is unlikely, because shorter telomeres and telomerase inactivation is more often associated with increased cancer rates, and the mortality from cancer occurs late in life.

In humans, shorter telomeres were associated with poorer health and aging and were also observed in preneoplastic stages, supporting a role for this mechanism in generating genomic aberrations in oncogenesis [57–60]. The model for gene amplification due to telomere abnormalities and the break at fragile sites (discussed below) was first described in maize and results from the breakage/fusion/bridge (B/F/B) cycles [61]. B/F/B cycles are initiated when broken ends of chromosomes fuse, resulting in a dicentric chromosome. During anaphase, the two centromeres are pulled in opposite directions and the dicentric chromosome generates a chromosome with an inverted duplication of terminal sequences to break. The B/F/B cycle continues in the next cell cycle because this chromosome also has broken ends. The B/F/B cycles were observed like primary mechanism for gene amplification in hamster cells [62].

In human cancer, evidence of B/F/B cycles was provided by the high frequency of anaphase bridges in early passage tumor cells and tumors [63, 64]. On the other hand, it was proven that human tumor cells in culture presenting gene amplification contain DM chromosomes, and the clones with low-copy amplification contained structures related to B/F/B cycles [65, 66]. There are evidences that B/F/B cycles may generate amplicons. These results were obtained by cytogenetic analyses of HSRs in tumor cell lines and in model systems with amplifications following drug treatments [67, 68]. The model explains that loss of the DNA sequences distal to the gene under selection or their translocation to another chromosome is also possible.

HSR may arise from the integration or fusion of double minute with a chromosome [50]. Currently, the data available suggests that fusion and reintegration constitute a pathway for the evolution of extrachromosomal elements, but the site of HSR insertion has never been characterized at a nucleotide resolution [50].

3.2. Fragile sites

Fragile sites are part of normal chromosome structures existing in each individual and represent chromosome regions that are late in replicating and prone to breakage under conditions of replication stress. Fragile sites occur after partial inhibition of DNA synthesis and are constituted in regions presenting site-specific gaps and breaks on metaphase chromosomes. Common fragile sites are normally stable in somatic cells, but it was observed that following treatment of cultured cells with replication inhibitors, fragile sites display gaps, breaks, rearrangements [69, 70]. Fragile sites extend over large regions of high DNA flexibility and are associated with genes.

The molecular nature and mechanisms involved in fragile site instability was unknown till recently. In many cancer cells, fragile sites and associated genes suffer frequent deletions and/or rearrangement, demonstrating their role in genome instability during the oncogenesis process. As a group, fragile sites are heterogeneous and seem to extend over broad regions 0.3–9-Mb long. The regions comprising fragile site are particularly associated with a high frequency of recombinogenic events, including co-localization with chromosome aberrations sites related to various cancers [69].

Accordingly to several studies, there are around 127 known fragile sites in the human genome, defined as "common" or "rare" based on their frequency [71, 72]. Common fragile sites (CFSs) are a normal part of the human genome and are typically replicative stable [73]. CFSs are not the result of nucleotide repeat expansion mutations. The majority of breakages at CFSs are further distinguished depending on their sensitivity to the drugs used to induce their expression (e.g., low doses of the antibiotic aphidocilin (APH)) [74].

The breakage effect of APH may be reduced by using a co-treatment with low concentrations of the topoisomerase I inhibitor and camptothecin (CPT) [75]. CFS regions are highly conserved in vertebrate species, including mouse and primates [76–78]. CFSs initiate proper replication but slow to complete it, introducing breaks from unreplicated regions of DNA [79]. The mechanism proposed for CFS instability resides in this late replication. Late replication may occur due to formation of non-B DNA structures such as hairpins and toroids that block the replication fork in AT rich regions [80].

Rare fragile sites (RFSs) are classified into two sub-groups based on the compounds that induce breakage, folate-sensitive groups and nonfolate-sensitive groups, which are sensitive at bromodeoxyuridine (BrdU) or distamycin A, an antibiotic that binds to AT-pairs of the DNA sequence. The folate-sensitive group is characterized by an expansion of CGG repeats, while the nonfolate-sensitive group contains many AT-rich minisatellite repeats [81–83]. The genome instability mechanism of CGG and AT-rich repeats characteristic for RFSs can form DNA structure (hairpins and other non-B DNA) replication forks, leading to breakage [84, 85]. On the other hand, it was demonstrated that DNA polymerase stops at CTG and CGG triplet repeat sequences, which can result in continuous DNA synthesis via slippage [79].

Fragile site regions are stable in normal cells and become unstable in tumor cells. The breakage of the fragile sites may be caused by mutations leading to a blockage of replication, or by a cell cycle perturbation and gene involved in the DNA repair process deregulation [86]. Several reports developed the concepts that underlie the mechanisms leading to fragile site expression and chromosomal rearrangements at fragile sites in tumors. The analysis of DNA damage response in various tumor types, including bladder, breast, colorectal, and lung tumors, found that early stages of cancer development are associated with an active DNA damage response, including phosphorylated ATR (ataxia telangiectasia and Rad3-related protein), ATM (ataxia telangiectasia mutated), CHK1 (checkpoint kinases), CHK2 kinases, phosphorylated histone H2AX, and p53 [87-88].

These events are linked to a high frequency of LOH (loss of heterozygoty) at known fragile site regions. The explained mechanisms sustained that in precancerous lesions, the blockage or collapsed replication leads to ATR activation and with subsequent DNA double strand breaks. Tumor cells that escape apoptosis or cell cycle arrest will exhibit allelic imbalances, especially at target fragile sites because of replication sensitivity. Further, the model sustains the necessity of p53 mutation and/or other genes involved in checkpoints control, leading therefore to cancer progression. Lesions at common fragile sites are indicators of replication stress during early stages of tumorigenesis [70].

Fragile sites regions are targets for the initiation of the amplification process due to breakage. Several studies showed that boundaries of some amplicons generated through the amplification process mapped to common chromosomal fragile sites in hamster cells [89–90]. Evidences of the role of fragile sites in human cancer regarding gene amplification are scarce. One example of cell line model is for the *MET* amplicons in the esophageal adenocarcinoma map within the fragile site FRA7G [91].

Aphidicolin-sensitive fragile sites FRA5D, FRA5F, and FRA5C, which map distal to dihydrofolate reductase gene (*DHFR)* on 5q, are infrequently expressed and are less likely to contribute to the amplification process. In order for the gene amplification process to take effect the target gene must be in the close proximity of fragile sites, similar to the *MET* amplicon. The breakage at specific genomic sites may not contribute to the amplification process, and no evidence of recurrent amplicon boundaries was found using array CGH in a human cell culture system [92].

3.3. Amplified genes in cancer

The amplification process is important for deciphering oncogenesis molecular biology, prognosis, and targeted therapies. A good example of gene amplification is dihydrofolate reductase gene (*DHFR*), which usually occurs during progression of methotrexate-resistant acute lymphoblastic leukemia [93]. In cancer, the most amplified genes are members of four different oncogene families: *MYC*, cyclin D1 (or *CCND1*), *EGFR*, and *RAS*. The amplified DNA segment usually involves several hundred kilobases and can contain many genes.

In breast cancer, *MYC, ERBB2, CCND1, EGFR*, or *MDM2* were found to be amplified concomitantly [94]. Moreover, it has been reported that there is a direct correlation between the number of amplifications and an advanced breast cancer and poor survival [95]. *MYC* oncogene is amplified in many types of cancer such as small-cell lung cancer, breast cancer, esophageal cancer, cervical cancer, ovarian cancer, and head and neck cancer [96].

Among the best-known oncogenes that are amplified in cancer cells is *N-MYC*. This gene codes for a transcription factor that plays a physiologic role in stimulating cellular proliferation and is commonly amplified in neuroblastoma where patients have poor clinical prognosis. Amplification of *N-MYC* in neuroblastoma has a valuable prognostic significance, and is correlated with an advanced tumor stage [97], along with *MYC* and *ERBB2* in breast cancer [94].

In malignant thyroid tumors, *C-MYC* gene overexpression and amplification has also been correlated with tumor aggressiveness [98]. Overexpression of cyclins is also an important element in thyroid oncogenesis, playing a crucial role in PTC pathogenesis [98]. *CCND1*, a cell cycle key regulator of G1/S transition, is a frequent target of mutagenesis in many tumors; amplification and rearrangement of its gene can lead to the over-production of this cell cycle regulatory protein. *CCND1* amplification also occurs in breast, esophageal, hepatocellular, and head and neck cancer [99].

EGFR (*ERBB1*) is amplified in glioblastoma and head and neck cancer. Amplification of *ERBB2* (also called *HER2/neu*) in breast cancer correlates with a poor prognosis. A monoclonal antibody against the product of this oncogene (trastuzumab) is effective in breast cancers that overexpress HER2/neu.

New data were acquired using array-CGH technique, bringing to knowledge the complex aspect of oncogene amplification in cancer. Using array-CGH analysis on identification of an 8p12 amplicon in anaplastic thyroid carcinoma (ATC) cell lines, six genes were found to be amplified, *DUSP26,MET, MYC, PVT1, YAP1* and *CIAP1* [100]. *DUSP26* effectively dephosphorylates *p38* and formed a physical complex with *p38*, promoting the survival of ATC cells by inhibiting *p38*-mediated apoptosis.

The *AIB1* oncogene is located on chromosome 20q, a region frequently amplified and overexpressed in breast cancer [101–102]. High levels of *AIB1* mRNA or protein predict significantly worse prognosis and overall survival in breast cancer patients [103]. *AIB1* is a transcriptional co-activator that promotes the transcriptional activity of multiple nuclear receptors such as the estrogen and progesterone receptors [104].

In cervical cancer, the array-CGH technique revealed that the 3q26.3 amplification was the most consistent chromosomal aberration in primary tissues of cervical carcinoma, and an increased copy number of *PIK3CA* gene was identified [105]. *PIK3CA* is known to be involved in the PI 3-kinase/AKT signaling pathway, which plays an important role in regulating cell growth and apoptosis.

In pancreatic cancer, chromosome 19q13 was found amplified containing *PAK4* gene [106]. *PAK* proteins are critical effectors that link *Rho GTPases* to cytoskeleton reorganization and nuclear signaling. *PAK4* interacts specifically with the GTP-bound form of *Cdc42Hs* and weakly activates the *JNK* family of *MAP* kinases. *PAK4* gene is not in a mutated oncogenic form but the activation of the *PAK4* gene promotes *KRAS2* gene mutation, a very frequent event in pancreatic cancer [106].

DNA amplification represents an important mechanism during human multistep hepatocarcinogenesis. Several genes were found to be amplified within 1q21 amplicon in hepatocellular carcinoma: *CREB3L4* (cyclic AMP responsive element binding protein3-like 4); *JTB* (Jumping Translocation Breakpoint) is a transmembrane protein that suffers an unbalanced translocation in various types of cancers [107]; *INTS3* and *SNAPAP,* whose role in oncogenesis remains to be defined; *SHC1* is involved in signal transduction from receptor tyrosine kinases to downstream signal to *RAS* [108–109]; *CKS1B* (CDC28 protein kinase regulatory subunit 1B), Cks1 expression was closely associated with poor differentiation and also negatively associated with $p27^{kip1}$ in hepatocellular carcinoma [110]; *CHD1L* (Chromodomain Helicase/ATPase DNA Binding Protein 1-Like, also known as Amplified in Liver Cancer 1, *ALC1*) whose increased expression was associated with clinicopathological features such as microsatellite tumor formation, venous infiltration, and advanced tumor stage, overall survival time, and the disease-free survival rate [111]. Moreover, *Glyoxalase 1 (Glo1)* gene aberrations are associated with tumorigenesis and progression in numerous cancers. Hepatocarcinoma cells with genetic amplified Glo1 gene express higher levels of Glo1 and are more sensitive to cell killing effects if Glo1 expression is down-regulated [112]. The study supports the potential of Glo1 as therapeutic target in patients with hepatocellular carcinoma and genetic Glo1 amplification.

Human oncogene *JUN* gene amplification/overexpression was found in highly aggressive sarcomas and in hepatocellular carcinomas, along with amplification/overexpression of MAP3K5. *JUN* overexpression could interfere with adipocytic differentiation and promote angiogenesis [113, 114].

Amplification of the *FGFR2* gene was identified in a subset of Chinese and Caucasian patients with gastric cancer. Fibroblast growth factor receptor family members (*FGFR1–4*) belong to the *RTK* superfamily. Through interaction with FGF ligands, the receptors are involved in diverse cellular functions including regulation of development processes, mediation of cell proliferation, and differentiation, as well as angiogenesis and tissue regeneration [115, 116]. FGF ligand binding leads to kinase activation and downstream signaling to phosphoinositide 3-kinase (PI3K)-AKT and mitogen-activated protein kinase–extracellular signal–regulated kinase (MAPK-ERK) pathways [117]. Genetic modifications or overexpression of FGFRs have been associated with tumorigenesis and progression in breast, prostate, stomach, and hematologic malignancies [118, 119]. *FGFR2* amplification leads to constitutive activation of the FGFR2 signaling pathway in gastric cancer, and furthermore inhibition of this pathway using a well-tolerated, potent, and selective inhibitor can lead to rapid and durable tumor regressions in *FGFR2*-amplified gastric cancer xenograft models, representing an important treatment target [120].

3.4. Chromosomal translocations

Chromosomal translocations (CTs) are very common in human cancer, and the molecular mechanisms involved are complex and poorly understood. CTs are involved in several types of cancer, particularly in hematopoietic and lymphoid tumors [121]. This type of chromosomal abnormality seems to provide a selective growth advantage for some stem or progenitor cells, which may further initiate the development of some malignant tumors. In case of oncogenes, CTs may change the original locations of proto-oncogenes, generating effects on the gene products through two major ways [122, 123]. One is to generate oncogenic fusion proteins and the other way is that proto-oncogenes are brought into proximity with regulatory elements, causing the overexpression of proto-oncogene.

The first specific chromosomal translocation identified in human cancer was the Philadelphia chromosome [t(9;22)], which underlies chronic myeloid leukemia (CML). The fusion of chromosomes 9 and 22 leads to the joining of two unrelated genes, the *C-ABL* gene, which encodes a tyrosine kinase and is located on chromosome 9, and the gene *BCR* (for breakpoint recombination) located on chromosome 22.10 [124]. A chimeric protein (BCR-ABL) with novel transforming properties is formed from this specific chromosomal rearrangement. BCR-ABL oncoprotein has an abnormal tyrosine kinase activity and is associated with the tumorigenesis of CML and acute lymphoblastic leukemia (ALL) [124]. Duplication of the Philadelphia chromosome leads to accelerated CML blast phase, suggesting that increased copies of this aberrant gene confer a dose-dependent transforming effect [125]. Similar to t(9;22) in acute promyelocytic leukemia (APL), a chromosomal rearrangement joins a novel gene t(15;17), resulting in the formation of promyelocytic leukemia-retinoic acid receptor α (*PML-RAR*α) fusion oncoprotein [126].

PML-RAR function is unknown, but this translocation underlies the response of this leukemia type to treatment with trans-retinoic acid. Another intergenic, CT t(12;21), leads to a novel chromosomal translocation product, *TEL-AML1*, which requires a specific treatment for pediatric acute lymphoblastic leukemia [127].

A classic example is the overexpression of proto-oncogene c-MYC in Burkitt lymphoma due to t(8;14) that results in *c-MYC* gene juxtaposed to immunoglobulin heavy chain (IGH) regulatory elements [128, 129]. Further expression of the gene is directed by the strong immunoglobulin heavy-chain enhancer, which is constitutively active in B lymphocytes. Thus, c-*MYC* overexpression is a potent force driving cellular proliferation.

The t(11;14) translocation juxtaposes *CCND1* and immunoglobulin enhancer elements and is characteristic of mantle-cell lymphoma. The t(11;14) translocation juxtaposes *CCND1* and immunoglobulin enhancer elements [130].

The ability to grow leukemic cells in culture long enough to allow cytogenetic analysis has facilitated the characterization of chromosomal translocations in leukemia. However, specific chromosomal translocations have also been observed in solid tumors. Aside from interchromosomal translocations, intrachromosomal translocations are also associated with cancer. Around 60–70% of PTCs have a characteristic inv(10)(q11.2q21). The breakpoint is represented by *RET* gene locus (10q11.2), which is relegated to the opposite breakpoint of the *H4* (D10S170) or *NCOA4* (ELE1) gene (10q21) in the same chromosome [131]. The H4 protein is widely expressed in the nucleus and cytoplasm and its function is unknown [132]. In PTC, many types of rearrangement loci (11 rearranged forms) were noted and PTC1(H4, CCDC6)-RET and PTC3(NCOA4)-RET are the most common [133]. PTC2-RET is a less common type of PTC-RET [134]. These rearrangements can lead to constitutively ligand-independent RET activity involved in thyroid carcinogenesis. The hypothesis sustain that the distances between RET and H4 loci are 18 Mb, therefore chromosome folding may close the two loci to each other in thyroid cells, increasing the probability of recombination between them in the interphase nuclei. This chromosomal folding is specific for thyroid cells, and this may explain why inv(10)(q11.2q21) is frequently seen in PTC [135].

It has been shown that in prostate carcinomas, the fusion between *TMPR552* gene and two transcription factors *ERG*1 or *ETV1* creates a fusion protein that increases proliferation and inhibits apoptosis of cells in the prostate gland, thereby facilitating their transformation into cancer cells [1].

The translocations of ETS are often found in human cancer, such as Ewing sarcoma [136–137], leukemia [138–139], prostate cancer [140], and breast cancer [141]. These once disparate tumors are now defined by a chromosomal translocation fusing the EWS gene to a number of transcription factors of the ETS gene family (the most common chimeric protein is EWS-FLI1) [142]. This chimeric product presumably acts directly on target promoters to direct the expression of genes that induce cellular proliferation. Identification of EWS translocations allowed the molecular grouping of a class of tumors whose proliferation is driven by similar genetic alterations and that respond to similar chemotherapeutic regimens.

4. Oncogene hypomethylation

The first epigenetic modification observed in human cancer was the loss of DNA methylation at the 5'citosine level (m5C residues replaced by unmethylated C residues), reported in 1983 [143]. This discovery was often regarded as an unwelcome complication, and all of the attention was focused on the opposite effect hypermethylation of promoters of genes that are silenced in cancers (e.g., tumor-suppressor genes). Global hypomethylation of DNA in cancer was found associated especially with repeated DNA elements; this modification did not represent a research direction for many years [144]. However, changes in the pattern of DNA methylation have been a consistent modification in cancer cells. Both hypo- and hypermethylation were observed at various loci, but at this moment it is clear that DNA methylation plays an important role in carcinogenesis.

New deep sequencing methylome analyses have shown much more cancer-linked hypomethylation of unique gene sequences and hypermethylation of repeated sequences than previously found [145–148]. Targeting DNA repetitive sequence, DNA hypomethylation may induce genomic instability and mutation events in cancer genomes [149–152] by altering the intranuclear positioning of chromatin enhancing recombination [153–155] and activating retroviral elements [156]. Promoter hypomethylation of some genes may be associated with the development of cancer by regulating the activity of genes [157].

4.1. Genomic hypomethylation profiles in cancer

DNA methylation principally occurs at 5' cytosine from dinucleotide CpG sites [158, 159]. CpG dinucleotides are found in C+G-rich regions in the genome termed CpG islands, localized frequently at promoter or gene regulatory level. However, the vast majority of CpG dinucleotides are localized within the intergenic and intronic regions of the DNA, particularly within repeat sequences and transposable elements. Unmethylated CpG islands at gene level are associated with gene transcription. In normal somatic cells, between 70% and 90% of CpG dinucleotides are methylated, which constitute approximately 0.75–1% of the total number of bases in the genome, while most CpG islands are unmethylated [160]. A part of genes promoter region are methylated as part of normal developmental processes or tissue specific (e.g., germline specific genes-MAGE genes) [161]. In X chromosomes in female dosage compensation (imprinted genes of X chromosomes in females), where only one of two copies is active, methylation of regulatory regions is involved in the repression of the expression of the silent loci [162].

Recently, high-resolution genome-wide analyses of DNA methylation changed the idea that considers oncogenesis being characterized predominantly of hypomethylated DNA repeats and hypermethylated gene regions [163–164]. The hallmark for cancer is represented by global losses of DNA methylation with local hypermethylation and hypomethylation of specific genes [165–167].

Evaluation of the majority of cancers showed that a major contributor to global DNA hypomethylation is hypomethylation of tandem and interspersed DNA repeats [165, 168]. Several studies using CpG methylation-sensitive restriction endonucleases or sodium bisulfite reported that hypomethylation was often found at gene sequence level (including metastasis-associated genes) [157, 165].

4.2. Hypomethylation of DNA repeats sequence in cancer

Repeat sequences are represented by transposable elements found interspersed throughout the genome, or simple repeat sequences, such as DNA satellites, found in pericentromeric or subtelomeric region of chromosomes. These are normally methylated within the healthy genome [169].

In cancer, hypomethylation of DNA repeats is a result of the demethylation process rather than the preexisting hypomethylation in a cancer stem cell [170]. The frequency of cancer-associated hypomethylation of DNA repeats is dependent with disease progression (tumor grade, stage) [171, 172]. Hypomethylation is also seen in tumor adjacent tissues and in benign tumors (breast fibroadenomas and ovarian cystadenomas), but at a lower level than cancer [145, 165, 173, 174].

Hypomethylation may affect transcription and hypomethylation of interspersed DNA repeats within promoter modifies the chromatin boundaries resulting in transcription activation of nearby genes [175, 176]. Along with the effects upon transcription, hypomethylation can affect alternative splicing and hypomethylation of a minor portion of interspersed DNA repeats may occasionally cause induction of retroviral element transcription [156]. Several studies reported numerous evidences for the causal relationships between DNA hypomethylation and increased transcription as well as hypomethylation and cancer [177–179].

Regions of cancer-associated changes in DNA methylation are found in short interspersed or clustered regions, as well as in long blocks [180–182]. Dante et al. described hypomethylation of LINE-1 (a highly repeated interspersed repeat) in mononuclear cells from patients with chronic lymphocytic leukemia [183]. Along with hypomethylation of LINE-1, Alu repeats were also subsequently observed hypomethylated in many other types of cancers [183–186]. In breast adenocarcinomas, ovarian epithelial cancers, and Wilms tumors, a hypomethylation of centromeric and juxtacentromeric satellite DNA was noted [173, 174, 187]. Moreover, another classes of tandem repeats (macrosatellite DNAs) and segmental duplications were found hypomethylated in various cancers [188–190]. The loss of DNA methylation in cancer varies according to the tumor type and subclasses of DNA repeat [191–193].

Gathering the result of the presented studies, we may conclude that in many types of cancer, hypomethylation of DNA repeats represents a highly informative prognostic marker and/or predictor of survival [194–197].

4.3. Hypomethylation of DNA gene enhancer sequence in cancer

Gene expression levels may be further modulated by DNA methylation levels at upstream enhancer sites [198], which can affect the binding of transcription factors at (CpG) islands [199]. In normal cells, DNA demethylation at enhancer's level is correlated with upregulation of expression of the associated gene. It was shown that the binding of FoxA1/FOXA1 transcriptional factors to enhancers is inhibited by DNA methylation at the respective binding site [200]. In this case, modification of DNA methylation status (demethylation) at the enhancer level may lead to an open chromatin state allowing the access of transcription factors at the active enhancer [201–202]. Following DNA demethylation, FoxD3 transcription factor binds at the enhancer level, allowing the recruitment of FoxA1 and conversion of the enhancer to a state that is set for activity. Local DNA demethylation leads also to changes in histone H3K27 or H3K9 methylation [200]. FOXA1 is an important factor for oncogenesis being involved in various types of cancer [203]. Thus, DNA hypomethylation from transcription regulatory regions may cause changes in expression [204].

4.4. Genomic hypomethylation in promoters and within gene bodies

Hypomethylation of transcription regulatory regions is less frequent than hypermethylation of CpG island promoters in cancer. Some of the gene regions (including transcription control sequences) were associated with loss of DNA methylation. Currently, there are data that sustain that promoter hypomethylation of some genes may be associated with the development of cancer, regulating the activity of genes [157]. For example, promoter hypomethylation of specific immunity-related genes (e.g., cytokine IL-10) may activate the specific gene expression to inhibit the immune response in breast cancer [205], and the promoter hypomethylation of SPAN-Xb, an immunogenic antigen, can induce de novo B-cell response in myeloma cells [206]. However, the biological significance of promoter hypomethylation in cancer is still poorly understood [144]. Hypomethylation of gene promoters must cooperate with other key activators such as transcriptional factors to control gene expression [207, 208].

Promoters may overlap tissue-specific (T-DMR) or cancer-specific (C-DMR) differentially methylated DNA regions [209]. Most of the non-imprinted, autosomal T-DMR promoters are not the main type of vertebrate DNA promoters, and the genes presenting T-DMR promoters become activated after experimentally induced demethylation 5-deoxyazacytidine [209].

Intragenic epigenetic marks have been also involved in normal gene expression regulation and inverse relationships between imprinted gene expression and DNA methylation level was observed [210]. T-DMR regions were found not only inside many genes, but also in downstream promoters, flanking certain subsets of genes [211, 212]. Moreover, besides first exon, T-DMRs are also present at exonic and intronic sequences, insulators, intragenic ncRNA genes, and 3 'terminal regions [213, 214].

The role of these regions is to connect DNA and chromatin, inducing tissue-specific chromatin epigenetic marks inside genes [215, 216]. This relationship between DNA and chromatin modification at gene level may help determine alternative promoter usage, modulate the rate of transcription initiation or elongation, and direct the choice of alternative splice sites [217, 218]. For moderately expressed genes, DNA methylation level in the middle of the gene is correlated with higher transcription rates, being related to nucleosome positioning [219]. In genes with CpG-poor promoters, methylated sequences located downstream binds Polycomb repressor complexes [212], which are being associated with repression of promoters [220].

On the other hand, certain histone modifications may direct the choice of splice junction through direct interactions with proteins that mark exon–intron junctions, altering rates of transcription and nucleosome positioning [221, 222]. As we mentioned before, DNA methylation may also be involved in regulating alternative splicing, intron–exon junctions being enriched in sharp transitions in DNA methylation levels [223] (e.g., malignant prostate cancer cells have enrichment of DNA hypermethylation at exon–intron junctions [224]). Therefore, these findings highlight the involvement of DNA methylation levels in determining alternative splicing in tumor cells, suggesting that cancer-associated DNA hypomethylation in intronic and exonic sequences can modulate the amount and type of gene products and thereby contribute to tumor formation or progression.

TGFB2 gene contains an intronic Alu repeat that was found hypomethylated in some cancer cell lines. Their hypomethylation at this site might be related to the significant upregulation of *TGFB2* gene, being an example of cancer-associated hypomethylation and a target chromatin associated epigenetic changes [225]. *PRDM16* presents gene-body hypomethylation (overlapping an exon) in some of the cancer cell lines, whereas *NOTCH2* also showed gene-body hypomethylation (in a subregion of repetitive DNA).

Gene encoding the protease urokinase (*PLAU/uPA*) is overexpressed and was found hypomethylated along with tumor progression in breast cancers and prostate cancers [157]. Also, other genes were observed to display hypomethylation and transcriptional activation in cancer, *S100A4*, mesothelin, claudin4, trefoil factor 2, maspin, *PGP9.5*, *POMC*, and the heparinase gene [144].

DNA hypomethylation is closely associated with morphological dedifferentiation in thyroid cancers. Four oncogenes (*INSL4*, *DPPA2*, *TCL1B* and *NOTCH4*) were frequently regulated by hypomethylation in anaplastic and medulary carcinoma [226].

Hematopoietin, *TNF*, *IL1*, *IL10*, and *IL17* families of cytokines had a significant tendency to be hypomethylated in five cancer types (colon, kidney, stomach, lung, and breast) [227].

Hypomethylation and increased expression in cancer has been shown for *R-RAS* [228]. A strong association of *CDH3* promoter demethylation and *P-cadherin* expression evident with histological grade and invasiveness in breast cancer was observed [229]. In Stage III and IV gastric cancer *cyclin D*2 activation is associated with promoter demethylation, activation of *synuclein* γ is associated with progression and metastatic potential in a range of solid tumors, and *maspin* expression in colorectal cancer is associated with microsatellite unstable tumors [230–232].

Hypomethylation and overexpression of some imprinted genes, including the *IGF-II*and *H19* genes, are implicated in carcinogenesis [233–235].

The putative oncogene, *ELMO3*, is overexpressed in non-small cell lung cancer in combination with hypomethylation of its promoter and these cancer-specific events are associated with the formation of metastases [236].

Aberrant hypomethylation and overexpression of *WNT5A* may be functionally important in the progression of prostate cancer. Along with *WNT5A*, *S100P*, and *CRIP1*, which have been previously implicated in cancer progression, are also regulated at the transcriptional level in prostate cancer by hypomethylation [237].

Evidence is accumulating for the biological significance and clinical relevance of DNA hypomethylation in cancer and for cancer-linked demethylation, and those seem to be highly dynamic processes.

5. MicroRNA genes

At present, a special consideration is given to small non-coding RNA molecules (microRNA) to their functions and involvement in human diseases. There are an extensive number of studies that link microRNA alterations to cancer pathogenesis. MicroRNA genes encode for a single RNA strand of about 21 to 23 nucleotides, which regulate gene expression by specifically targeting certain mRNAs in order to prevent them from coding for a specific protein. Some microRNA genes are mapped in chromosomal regions that undergo rearrangements, deletions, and amplifications in cancer. A growing amount of data demonstrates that microRNA genes display a different pattern of expression in various malignancies; they are found up-regulated or down-regulated and therefore can function either as oncogenes activating the malignant transformation (by down-regulating tumor-suppressor genes), or as tumor-suppressor genes blocking the malignant transformation (by down-regulating oncogenes). In numerous types of cancers, many different microRNA have been shown to act as oncogenes, their expression profiling presenting specific signatures associated with malignant transformation. Cancer-associated microRNA molecules are also called oncomir (oncomiR).

The first microRNA that has been proven to act as oncogene in human cancer was *miR-17/92* polycistronic cluster known as *OncomiR-1*, which comprises six microRNAs: *miR-17, miR-18a, miR-19a, miR-20a, miR-19b-1, and miR-92a-1* [238]. The *miR-17/92* cluster is located in the locus of intron 3 of *C13orf25* gene at 13q31.3, in a region frequently amplified in several types of lymphomas and solid tumor. It has been shown that the locus is amplified and overexpressed in human B cell lymphomas, malignant lymphoma cell lines and in lung cancers especially with small-cell lung cancer histology [239, 240]. Insertional mutagenesis studies using retroviruses indicates that *miR-17/92* acts as an oncogene in T cell lymphomas; it was shown that soon after SL3-3 murine leukemia virus infection, mice developed tumors if provirus integrates into the proximity of the gene encoding *miR-17/92* cistron [241]. Moreover, other studies uncovered that *C-MYC* and *E2F3* gene products may induce *miR-17/92* polycistronic expression through direct binding to the cluster promoter. Two microRNAs belonging to the cluster, *miR-17-5p* and *miR-20a* negatively regulate *E2F1* activity, which confirms that the *miR-17/92* can promote cell proliferation through the exchange of *E2F1* to *E2F3* pro-apoptotic proliferative [242]. Thus, *miR-17/92* represents an anti-apoptotic oncogene and *miR-20a* inhibition using antisense oligonucleotides can induce apoptosis after treatment with doxorubicin [243].

Along with the *miR-17/92* cluster from the *miR-17* family, two other paralogue miRNA gene clusters are produced, *miR-106b/25* and *miR-106a/363*, which possess oncogenic potential and are known to be involved in wide types of cancers. The *miR-106b/25* cluster is located in intron 13 of the minichromosome maintenance complex component 7 (*MCM7*) oncogene at 7q22.1 and it contains the following three miRNAs: *miR-106b, miR-93,* and *miR-25*. Recently, findings sustain the oncogenic potential of this cluster and reports correlate *miR-106b/25* member expression levels with processes such as tumor growth, cell survival, and angiogenesis [244, 245]. The oncogenic potential of the *miR-106b/25* cluster in malignant transformation is achieved by targeting and down-regulation of several tumor-suppressor genes such as *p21, E2F1,* and *PTEN* [246–248]. Furthermore, other recent work suggests that in breast cancer cells, *miR-106b/25* cluster overexpression leads to overcoming doxorubicin-induced senescence and cells become drug resistant through a mechanism that involves targeting *E-cadherin* transcriptional activators *EP300* [249]. The second cluster, *miR-106a/363,* is located on chromosome X (Xq26.2) and comprises of six miRNAs: *miR-106a, miR-18b, miR-20b, miR-19b-2, miR-92a-2, and miR-363.* A series of reports indicates an oncogenic potential for members of the cluster, for example *miR-106a* and *miR-92-2* were found overexpressed in colon and prostate cancer and also in leukemia and Ewing Sarcoma [250–252].

Another important oncomir is represented by *miR-155* found overexpressed in several malignancies: chronic lymphocytic leukemia (CLL), B cell lymphoma, Hodgkin's lymphoma or Burkitt's type, and breast cancer. Some reports have shown that clinical isolates from B cell lymphomas, including those with large cells, contain a number of copies of *miR-155,* about 30 times higher than normal B cells [253–256]. Also, results suggest that the pancreatic ductal adenocarcinomas overexpression of *miR-155* determined decreased levels of *TP53INP1* leading to apoptosis elusion and cell growth development [257].

A promising oncomir is also *miR-21,* one of the most common miRNA associated with human cancers. *MicroRNA-21* high expression has been found in a variety of cancers including breast cancer, brain malignant tumors, glioblastomas, pancreatic, colorectal, liver, gastric, lung, skin, thyroid, ovarian, esophagus, prostate, cervical, and different lymphatic and hematopoietic cancers [250, 258–263]. Elevated *miR-21* levels have been linked to cell proliferation, apoptosis reduction, and cell migration in neoplastic transformation; it has been found that this oncomir targets and down-regulates a number of tumor-suppressor genes including *PTEN, PDCD4, BCL2, RECK, JAG1, HNRPK, BTG2, TGFBRII,* and thus sustaining cancer's invasion and metastasis [264, 265]. Moreover, experiments using transfection of MCF-7 cell lines with anti-miR-21 oligonucleotide conducted to cell growth suppression in vitro and tumor growth in vivo had an increase of programmed cell death rate [266].

Altogether, these studies illustrate a major role for microRNA genes in cancer pathogenesis (Table 2); many of them have oncogenic activity and could represent valuable biomarkers very useful for cancer screening or assessment of the therapeutic effects of anti-cancer treatments.

MicroRNA	Cancer type	miRNA function	Potential targets	Reference
miR-21	Glioblastoma	Increase cell growth Inhibit apoptosis Promote cell cycle	*HNRNPK*I *TP63*	[267]

MicroRNA	Cancer type	miRNA function	Potential targets	Reference
	Breast	-	*RECK*I*TIMP3*	[268]
		Increase cell growth Increase metastasis	*PTEN*	[269, 270]
		Promote cell growth Promote cell migration Promote tumor growth	*ANKRD46*	[271]
		-	*PDCD4* *PTEN* *BCL2*	[272]
		Promote cell invasion Promote metastasis	*TPM1* *PDCD4* *SERPINB5*	[265]
	Cervix	Increase cell Proliferation Inhibit apoptosis Increase cell migration	*CCL20*	[273]
		Promote cell proliferation	*PDCD4*	[274]
	Prostate	Promote epithelial-mesenchymal transition	*BTG2*	[275]
		Induce tumor angiogenesis Activate AKT/ERK signaling		[276]
		Increase docetaxel resistance	*PDCD4*	[277]
		Promote cell proliferation Promote tumor growth		[278]
		Inhibit apoptosis Promote cell motility Promote cell invasion	*MARCKS*	[279]
	Blood	Promote cell migration Reduce apoptosis Promote cell growth	*PDCD4*	[280, 281]
miR-221 and 222	Prostate	Promote cell cycle G1/S transition Increase colony formation	*CDKN1B*	[282]
	Breast	Increase cell migration Increase cell invasion epithelial-mesenchymal transition	*TRPS1*	[283]

MicroRNA	Cancer type	miRNA function	Potential targets	Reference
		Increase tamoxifen resistance	*CDKN1B*	[284]
	Glioblastoma	Increase cell invasion	*TIMP3*	[285]
		Promote cell proliferation Promote cell invasion inhibit apoptosis	*GJA1*	[286]
	Thyroid	Promote cell transition to cell cycle S phase	*CDKN1B*	[287]
	Lung	Induce TRAIL resistance Increase cell migration	*PTEN* *TIMP3*	[288]
miR-155	Blood	Increase cell proliferation Increase clonogenity Inhibit apoptosis	*HDAC4*	[289]
		Promote PI3K-AKT signaling	*PIK3R1*	[290]
		Increase cell proliferation	*BCL2*	[291]
		Reduce cell cycle arrest	*SMAD5*	[292]
	Breast	Promote cell survival Induce chemoresistance Inhibit apoptosis	*FOXO3*	[293]
		Promote cell proliferation Promote tumor development	*SOCS1*	[294]
miR-17/92 cluster	Blood	Increase cell growth Increase cell cycle G1/S transition	*CDKN1A*	[295]
		Increase cell proliferation Increase imatinib - induced cell death		[296]
		Suppress apoptosis	*PTEN*	[297, 298]
	Retinoblastoma	Promote cell proliferation	*p21 and p57*	[299]
	Colon	Promote angiogenesis	*TSP-1* *CTGF*	[300]
	Breast		*ERa*	[301]
	Lung	Promote cell growth Reduce reactive oxygen species (ROS) generation	*HIF-1a*	[302]

MicroRNA	Cancer type	miRNA function	Potential targets	Reference
			HIF-1a, PTEN, BCL2L11, CDKNA and TSP-1.	[303,304]
miR-106b-25 cluster	Breast	Activate TGF-beta signaling Induce epithelial mesenchymal transition Induce a tumor initiating cell phenotype	*SMAD7*	[305]
	Gastric		*E2F1*	[306]
miR-191	Liver	Promote epithelial-mesenchymal transition Increase cell migration Increase cell invasion	*TIMP3*	[307]
		Promote cell proliferation Inhibit apoptosis Promote tumor growth		[308]
	Gastric		*NDST1*	[309]

(Source: OncomiRDB: http://bioinfo.au.tsinghua.edu.cn/member/jgu/oncomirdb/) [310].

Table 2. OncomiRs in human cancer

6. Concluding remarks

Oncogene activation by structural alteration (chromosomal rearrangement, gene fusion, mutation, and gene amplification) or epigenetic modification (gene promoter hypomethylation, microRNA expression pattern) confers an increased or a deregulated expression. Therefore, cells with such alterations possess a growth advantage or an increased survival rate. Given the fact that expression profiling of these alterations determines specific signatures associated with tumor classification, diagnosis, staging, prognosis and response to treatment, it highlights the importance of studying oncogenes activation mechanisms and the great potential that they hold as therapeutic tools in the near future.

Acknowledgements

This work was supported by Romanian Research Grant PCCA135/2012 and POSDRU/159/1.5 / S/135760

Author details

Anca Botezatu[1], Iulia V. Iancu[1], Oana Popa[2], Adriana Plesa[1], Dana Manda[2], Irina Huica[1], Suzana Vladoiu[2], Gabriela Anton[1] and Corin Badiu[3]

1 Molecular Virology, Stefan S. Nicolau Institute of Virology, Romania

2 Research Laboratory, "CI Parhon" National Institute of Endocrinology, Bucharest, Romania

3 Department of Endocrinology, "CI Parhon" National Institute of Endocrinology, Bucharest, Romania

References

[1] Tomlins SA, Rhodes DR, Perner S, Dhanasekaran SM, Mehra R, Sun XW, Varambally S, Cao X, Tchinda J, Kuefer R, Lee C, Montie JE, Shah RB, Pienta KJ, Rubin MA, Chinnaiyan AM. Recurrent fusion of TMPRSS2 and ETS transcription factor genes in prostate cancer. Science. 2005;310:644–8. DOI: 10.1126/science.1117679.

[2] Nakamura T, Mori T, Tada S, Krajewski W, Rozovskaia T, Wassell R, Dubois G, Mazo A, Croce CM, Canaani E. ALL-1 is a histone methyltransferase that assembles a supercomplex of proteins involved in transcriptional regulation. Mol Cell. 2002;10:1119–28. http://dx.doi.org/10.1016/S1097-2765(02)00740-2.

[3] Tsujimoto Y, Cossman J, Jaffe E, Croce CM. Involvement of the bcl-2 gene in human follicular lymphoma. Science. 1985;228:1440–3.

[4] Yeang CH, McCormick F, Levine A. Combinatorial patterns of somatic gene mutations in cancer. FASEB J. 2008;22(8):2605–22. DOI: 10.1096/fj.08-108985

[5] Rodenhuis S. RAS and human tumors. Semin Cancer Biol. 1992;3:241–7.

[6] Beaupre DM, Kurzrock R. RAS and leukemia: From basic mechanisms to gene-directed therapy. J Clin Oncol. 1999;17:1071–9.

[7] Kolch W. Meaningful relationships: The regulation of the Ras/Raf/MEK/ERK pathway by protein interactions. Biochemical Journal. 2000;351(2):289–305.

[8] Maldonado JL, Fridlyand J, Patel H, Jain AN, Busam K, Kageshita T, Ono T, Albertson DG, Pinkel D, Bastian BC. Determinants of BRAF mutations in primary melanomas. J Natl Cancer Inst. 2003;95:1878–90. DOI: 10.1093/jnci/djg123.

[9] Turri-Zanoni M, Medicina D, Lombardi D, Ungari M, Balzarini P, Rossini C, Pellegrini W, Battaglia P, Capella C, Castelnuovo P, Palmedo G, Facchetti F, Kutzner H, Nicolai P, Vermi W. Sinonasal mucosal melanoma: Molecular profile and therapeutic

implications from a series of 32 cases. Head Neck. 2013;35:1066–77. DOI: 10.1002/hed.23079.

[10] Colombino M, Capone M, Lissia A, Cossu A, Rubino C, De Giorgi V, Massi D, Fonsatti E, Staibano S, Nappi O, Pagani E, Casula M, Manca A, Sini M, Franco R, Botti G, Caracò C, Mozzillo N, Ascierto PA, Palmieri G. BRAF/NRAS mutation frequencies among primary tumors and metastases in patients with melanoma. J Clin Oncol. 2012;30(20):2522–2529. DOI: 10.1200/JCO.2011.41.2452.

[11] Long GV, Menzies AM, Nagrial AM, Haydu LE, Hamilton AL, Mann GJ, Hughes TM, Thompson JF, Scolyer RA, Kefford RF. Prognostic and clinicopathologic associations of oncogenic BRAF in metastatic melanoma. J Clin Oncol. 2011;29(10):1239–1246. DOI: 10.1200/JCO.2010.32.4327.

[12] Menzies AM, Haydu LE, Visintin L, Carlino MS, Howle JR, Thompson JF, Kefford RF, Scolyer RA, Long GV. Distinguishing clinicopathologic features of patients with V600E and V600K BRAF-mutant metastatic melanoma. Clin Cancer Res. 2012;18(12):3242–3249. DOI: 10.1158/1078-0432.CCR-12-0052.

[13] Burns PA, Jack A, Neilson F, Haddow S, Balmain A. Transformation of mouse skin endothelial cells in vivo by direct application of plasmid DNA encoding the human T24 H-ras oncogene. Oncogene. 1991;6:1973–8.

[14] Padua RA, Barrass NC, Currie GA. Activation of N-ras in a human melanoma cell line. Mol Cell Biol. 1985;5:582–5.

[15] Bucheit AD, Syklawer E, Jakob JA, Bassett RL Jr, Curry JL, Gershenwald JE, Kim KB, Hwu P, Lazar AJ, Davies MA. Clinical characteristics and outcomes with specific BRAF and NRAS mutations in patients with metastatic melanoma. Cancer. 2013;119(21):3821–3829. DOI: 10.1002/cncr.28306.

[16] Terheyden P, Houben R, Pajouh P, Thorns C, Zillikens D, Becker JC. Response to Imatinib Mesylate Depends on the Presence of the V559A-Mutated KIT Oncogene Journal of Investigative Dermatology. 2010;130:314–316. DOI: 10.1038/jid.2009.197.

[17] Beadling C, Jacobson-Dunlop E, Hodi FS, Le C, Warrick A, Patterson J, Town A, Harlow A, Cruz F 3rd, Azar S, Rubin BP, Muller S, West R, Heinrich MC, Corless CL. KIT gene mutations and copy number in melanoma subtypes. Clin Cancer Res. 2008;14:6821–8. DOI: 10.1158/1078-0432.CCR-08-0575.

[18] Minoo P, Moyer MP, Jass JR. Role of BRAF-V600E in the serrated pathway of colorectal tumourigenesis. Journal of Pathology. 2007;212(2):124–133. DOI: 10.1002/path.2160.

[19] Custodio A, Feliu J. Prognostic and predictive biomarkers for epidermal growth factor receptor-targeted therapy in colorectal cancer: Beyond KRAS mutations. Critical Reviews in Oncology/Hematology. 2013;85(1):45–81. DOI: 10.1016/j.critrevonc.2012.05.001.

[20] Diaz LA Jr, Williams RT, Wu J, Kinde I, Hecht JR, Berlin J, Allen B, Bozic I, Reiter JG, Nowak MA, Kinzler KW, Oliner KS, Vogelstein B. The molecular evolution of acquired resistance to targeted EGFR blockade in colorectal cancers. Nature. 2012;486(7404):537–540. DOI: 10.1038/nature11219.

[21] Zhu Z, Gandhi M, Nikiforova MN, Fischer AH, Nikiforov YE. Molecular profile and clinical-pathologic features of the follicular variant of papillary thyroid carcinoma. An unusually high prevalence of ras mutations. Am J Clin Pathol. 2003;120:71–7. DOI: 10.1309/ND8D9LAJTRCTG6QD.

[22] Vasko V, Ferrand M, Di Cristofaro J, Carayon P, Henry JF, de Micco C. Specific pattern of RAS oncogene mutations in follicular thyroid tumors. J Clin Endocrinol Metab. 2003;88:2745–52. DOI: http://dx.doi.org/10.1210/jc.2002-021186.

[23] Cohen Y, Xing M, Mambo E, Guo Z, Wu G, Trink B, Beller U, Westra WH, Ladenson PW, Sidransky D. BRAF mutation in papillary thyroid carcinoma. J Natl Cancer Inst. 2003;95:625–7. DOI: 10.1093/jnci/95.8.625.

[24] Davies H, Bignell GR, Cox C, Stephens P, Edkins S, Clegg S, Teague J, Woffendin H, Garnett MJ, Bottomley W, Davis N, Dicks E, Ewing R, Floyd Y, Gray K, Hall S, Hawes R, Hughes J, Kosmidou V, Menzies A, Paterson H, Marais R, Marshall CJ, Wooster R, Stratton MR, Futreal PA. Mutations of the BRAF gene in human cancer. Nature. 2002;417:949–54. DOI: 10.1038/nature00766.

[25] Xing M, Vasko V, Tallini G, Larin A, Wu G, Udelsman R, Ringel MD, Ladenson PW, Sidransky D. BRAF T1796A transversion mutation in various thyroid neoplasms. J Clin Endocrinol Metab. 2004;89:1365–8. DOI: http://dx.doi.org/10.1210/jc.2003-031488.

[26] Durante C, Puxeddu E, Ferretti E, Morisi R, Moretti S, Bruno R, Barbi F, Avenia N, Scipioni A, Verrienti A, Tosi E, Cavaliere A, Gulino A, Filetti S, Russo D. BRAF mutations in papillary thyroid carcinomas inhibit genes involved in iodine metabolism. J Clin Endocrinol Metab. 2007;92:2840–3. DOI: http://dx.doi.org/10.1210/jc.2006-2707.

[27] Cantwell-Dorris ER, O'Leary JJ, Sheils OM. BRAFV600E: Implications for carcinogenesis and molecular therapy. Mol Cancer Ther. 2011;10:385–94. DOI: 10.1158/1535-7163.MCT-10-0799.

[28] Gouveia C, Can NT, Bostrom A, Grenert JP, van Zante A, Orloff LA. Lack of association of BRAF mutation with negative prognostic indicators in papillary thyroid carcinoma: The University of California, San Francisco, experience. JAMA Otolaryngol Head Neck Surg. 2013;139:1164–70. DOI: 10.1001/jamaoto.2013.4501.

[29] Segouffin-Cariou C, Billaud M. Transforming ability of MEN2A-RET requires activation of the phosphatidylinositol 3-kinase/AKT signaling pathway. J Biol Chem. 2000;275:3568–7. DOI: 10.1074/jbc.275.5.3568.

[30] Raue F, Frank-Raue K. Update multiple endocrine neoplasia type 2. Fam Cancer. 2010;9:449–57. DOI: 10.1007/s10689-010-9320-2.

[31] Hedayati M, Zarif Yeganeh M, Sheikhol Eslami S, Rezghi Barez S, Hoghooghi Rad L, Azizi F. Predominant RET germline mutations in exons 10, 11, and 16 in Iranian patients with hereditary medullary thyroid carcinoma. J Thyroid Res. 2011;2011:264248. DOI: 10.4061/2011/264248.

[32] Machens A, Niccoli-Sire P, Hoegel J, Frank-Raue K, van Vroonhoven TJ, Roeher HD, Wahl RA, Lamesch P, Raue F, Conte-Devolx B, Dralle H. European Multiple Endocrine Neoplasia (EUROMEN) Study Group. Early malignant progression of hereditary medullary thyroid cancer.N Engl J Med. 2003;349:1517–2. DOI: 10.1056/NEJMoa012915.

[33] Figlioli G, Landi S, Romei C, Elisei R, Gemignani F. Medullary thyroid carcinoma (MTC) and RET proto-oncogene: Mutation spectrum in the familial cases and a meta-analysis of studies on the sporadic form. Mutat Res Rev Mutat Res. 2013;752:36–44. DOI: 10.1016/j.mrrev.2012.09.002.

[34] Marx SJ, Stratakis CA. Multiple endocrine neoplasia--introduction. J Intern Med. 2005;257:2–5. DOI: 10.1111/j.1365-2796.2004.01419.x.

[35] Eng C, Clayton D, Schuffenecker I, Lenoir G, Cote G, Gagel RF, van Amstel HK, Lips CJ, Nishisho I, Takai SI, Marsh DJ, Robinson BG, Frank-Raue K, Raue F, Xue F, Noll WW, Romei C, Pacini F, Fink M, Niederle B, Zedenius J, Nordenskjöld M, Komminoth P, Hendy GN, Mulligan LM. The relationship between specific RET proto-oncogene mutations and disease phenotype in multiple endocrine neoplasia type 2. International RET mutation consortium analysis. JAMA. 1996;276:1575–9. DOI: 10.1001/jama.1996.03540190047028.

[36] Mulligan LM, Eng C, Healey CS, Clayton D, Kwok JB, Gardner E, Ponder MA, Frilling A, Jackson CE, Lehnert H. Specific mutations of the RET proto-oncogene are related to disease phenotype in MEN 2A and FMTC. Nat Genet. 1994;6:70–74. DOI: 10.1038/ng0194-70.

[37] Kouvaraki MA, Shapiro SE, Perrier ND, Cote GJ, Gagel RF, Hoff AO, Sherman SI, Lee JE, Evans DB. RET proto-oncogene: A review and update of genotype-phenotype correlations in hereditary medullary thyroid cancer and associated endocrine tumors. Thyroid. 2005;15:531–44. DOI: 10.1089/thy.2005.15.531.

[38] Miyauchi A, Futami H, Hai N, Yokozawa T, Kuma K, Aoki N, Kosugi S, Sugano K, Yamaguchi K. Two germline missense mutations at codons 804 and 806 of the RET proto-oncogene in the same allele in a patient with multiple endocrine neoplasia type 2B without codon 918 mutation. Jpn J Cancer Res. 1999;90:15.

[39] Taketomi A1, Shirabe K, Muto J, Yoshiya S, Motomura T, Mano Y, Ikegami T, Yoshizumi T, Sugio K, Maehara Y. A rare point mutation in the Ras oncogene in hepatocellular carcinoma. Surg Today. 2013;43(3):289–92. DOI: 10.1007/s00595-012-0462-8.

[40] Rajagopalan H, Bardelli A, Lengauer C, Kinzler KW, Vogelstein B, Velculescu VE. RAF/RAS oncogenes and mismatch-repair status. Nature. 2002;418:934. DOI: 10.1038/418934a.

[41] Malats N, Porta M, Corominas JM, Piñol JL, Rifà J, Real FX. Ki-ras mutations in exocrine pancreatic cancer: Associations with clinicopathological characteristics and with tobacco and alcohol consumption. International Journal of Cancer. 1997;70:661–667. DOI: 10.1002/(SICI)1097-0215(19970317)70:6<661::AID-IJC6>3.0.CO;2-T.

[42] Agarwal A1, Saif MW. KRAS in pancreatic cancer. JOP. 2014;15(4):303–5. DOI: 10.6092/1590-8577/2660.

[43] Corcoran RB, Cheng KA, Hata AN, Faber AC, Ebi H, Coffee EM, Greninger P, Brown RD, Godfrey JT, Cohoon TJ, Song Y, Lifshits E, Hung KE, Shioda T, Dias-Santagata D, Singh A, Settleman J, Benes CH, Mino-Kenudson M, Wong KK, Engelman JA. Synthetic lethal interaction of combined BCL-XL and MEK inhibition promotes tumor regressions in KRAS mutant cancer models. Cancer Cell. 2013;23(1):121–128. DOI: 10.1016/j.ccr.2012.11.007.

[44] Wright AA, Howitt BE, Myers AP, Dahlberg SE, Palescandolo E, Van Hummelen P, MacConaill LE, Shoni M, Wagle N, Jones RT, Quick CM, Laury A, Katz IT, Hahn WC, Matulonis UA, Hirsch MS. Oncogenic mutations in cervical cancer: Genomic differences between adenocarcinomas and squamous cell carcinomas of the cervix. Cancer. 2013;119(21):3776–83. DOI: 10.1002/cncr.28288.

[45] Iida K, Nakayama K, Rahman MT, Rahman M, Ishikawa M, Katagiri A, Yeasmin S, Otsuki Y, Kobayashi H, Nakayama S, Miyazaki K. EGFR gene amplification is related to adverse clinical outcomes in cervical squamous cell carcinoma, making the EGFR pathway a novel therapeutic target. Br J Cancer. 2011;105(3):420–427. DOI: 10.1038/bjc.2011.22.

[46] Courtney KD, Corcoran RB, Engelman JA. The PI3K pathway as drug target in human cancer. J Clin Oncol. 2010;28(6):1075–1083. DOI: 10.1200/JCO.2009.25.3641.

[47] Schwarz JK, Payton JE, Rashmi R, Xiang T, Jia Y, Huettner P, Rogers BE, Yang Q, Watson M, Rader JS, Grigsby PW. Pathway-specific analysis of gene expression data identifies the PI3K/Akt pathway as a novel therapeutic target in cervical cancer. Clin Cancer Res. 2012;18(5):1464–1471. DOI: 10.1158/1078-0432.CCR-11-2485.

[48] Wahl GM, Robert de Saint Vincent B, DeRose ML. Effect of chromosomal position on amplification of transfected genes in animal cells. Nature. 1984;307:516–520.

[49] Albertson DG. Gene amplification in cancer. Trends Genet. 2006;22(8):447–55. DOI: http:// dx.doi.org /10.1016/j.tig.2006.06.007.

[50] Gibaud A, Vogt N, Brison O, Debatisse M, Malfoy B. Characterization at nucleotide resolution of the homogeneously staining region sites of insertion in two cancer cell lines. Nucleic Acids Res. 2013;41(17):8210–9. DOI: 10.1093/nar/gkt566.

[51] Windle BE, Wahl GM. Molecular dissection of mammalian gene amplification: New mechanistic insights revealed by analyses of very early events. Mutat. Res. 1992;276:199–224. DOI: 10.1016/0165-1110(92)90009-X.

[52] Eisenberg DTA. An evolutionary review of human telomere biology: The thrifty telomere hypothesis and notes on potential adaptive paternal effects. American Journal of Human Biology. 2011;23(2):149–167. DOI: 10.1002/ajhb.21127.

[53] Londono-Vallejo JA. Telomere length heterogeneity and chromosome instability. Cancer Lett. 2004;212(2):135–144. DOI: http://dx.doi.org/10.1016/j.canlet.2004.05.008.

[54] Sabatier L, Ricoul M, Pottier G, Murnane JP. The loss of a single telomere can result in instability of multiple chromosomes in a human tumor cell line. Mol. Cancer Res. 2005;3:139–150. DOI: 10.1158/1541-7786.MCR-04-0194.

[55] O'Hagan RC, Chang S, Maser RS, Mohan R, Artandi SE, Chin L, DePinho RA. Telomere dysfunction provokes regionalamplification and deletion in cancer genomes. Cancer Cell. 2002;2:149–155. DOI: http://dx.doi.org/10.1016/S1535-6108(02)00094-6.

[56] Chang S, Khoo C, DePinho RA. Modeling chromosomal instability and epithelial carcinogenesis in the telomerase-deficient mouse. Semin. Cancer Biol. 2001;11:227–239. DOI: 10.1006/scbi.2000.0374.

[57] Gisselsson D, Lv M, Tsao SW, Man C, Jin C, Höglund M, Kwong YL, Jin Y. Telomere-mediated mitotic disturbances in immortalized ovarian epithelial cells reproduce chromosomal losses and breakpoints from ovarian carcinoma. Genes Chromosomes Cancer. 2005;42:22–33. DOI: 10.1002/gcc.20094.

[58] Gisselsson D, Höglund M. Connecting mitotic instability and chromosome aberrations in cancer—can telomeres bridge the gap? Semin. Cancer Biol. 2005;15:13–23. DOI: 10.1016/j.semcancer.2004.09.002.

[59] Shen J, Gammon MD, Terry MB, Wang Q, Bradshaw P, Teitelbaum SL, Neugut AI, Santella RM. Telomere length, oxidative damage, antioxidants and breast cancer risk. Int J Cancer. 2009;124 (7):1637–43. DOI: 10.1002/ijc.24105.

[60] Cawthon RM, Smith KR, O'Brien E, Sivatchenko A, Kerber RA. Association between telomere length in blood and mortality in people aged 60 years or older. Lancet. 2003;361(9355):393–395. DOI: 10.1016/s0140-6736(03)12384-7.

[61] McClintock B. The stability of broken ends of chromosomes in Zea mays. Genetics. 1941;41:234–82.

[62] Toledo F, Buttin G, Debatisse M. The origin of chromosome rearrangements at early stages of AMPD2 gene amplification in Chinese hamster cells. Curr Biol. 1993;3:255–64. DOI: http://dx.doi.org/10.1016/0960-9822(93)90175-N.

[63] Londono-Vallejo JA. Telomere length heterogeneity and chromosome instability. Cancer Lett. 2004;212:135–144 41. DOI: http://dx.doi.org/10.1016/j.canlet.2004.05.008.

[64] Snijders AM, Fridlyand J, Mans DA, Segraves R, Jain AN, Pinkel D, Albertson DG. Shaping of tumor and drug-resistant genomes by instability and selection. Oncogene. 2003;22:4370–4379. DOI: 10.1038/sj.onc.1206482.

[65] Singer MJ, Mesner LD, Friedman CL, Trask BJ, Hamlin JL. Amplification of the human dihydrofolate reductase gene via double minutes is initiated by chromosome breaks. Proc Natl Acad Sci USA. 2000;97:7921–26. DOI: 10.1073/pnas.130194897.

[66] Lo AW, Sabatier L, Fouladi B, Pottier G, Ricoul M, Murnane JP. DNA amplification by breakage/fusion/bridge cycles initiated by spontaneous telomere loss in a human cancer cell line. Neoplasia. 2002;4(6):531–8. DOI: 10.1038/sj.neo.7900267.

[67] Ma K, Qiu L, Mrasek K, Zhang J, Liehr T, Quintana LG, Li Z. Common Fragile Sites: Genomic Hotspots of DNA Damage and Carcinogenesis. Int. J. Mol. Sci. 2012;13:11974–11999. DOI: 10.3390/ijms130911974.

[68] Murnane JP, Sabatier L. Chromosome rearrangements resulting from telomere dysfunction and their role in cancer. Bioessays. 2004;26:1164–1174. DOI: 10.1002/bies.20125.

[69] Glover TW, Arlt MF, Casper AM, Durkin SG. Mechanisms of common fragile site instability. Hum. Mol. Genet. 2005;2:R197–R205. DOI: 10.1093/hmg/ddi265.

[70] Glover TW. Common fragile sites. Cancer Lett. 2006;232(1):4–12. DOI: http://dx.doi.org/ 10.1016/ j.canlet. 2005.08.032.

[71] Lukusa T, Fryns JP. Human chromosome fragility. Biochimica et Biophysica Acta. 2008;1779(1):3–16. DOI: 10.1016/j.bbagrm.2007.10.005.

[72] Durkin SG, Glover TW. Chromosome fragile sites. Annual Review of Genetics. 2007;41:169–192. DOI: 10.1146/annurev.genet.41.042007.165900.

[73] Smith DI, Huang H, Wang L. Common fragile sites and cancer (review). International journal of oncology. 1998;12(1):187–96. DOI: 10.3892/ijo.12.1.187.

[74] Glover TW, Berger C, Coyle J, Echo B. DNA polymerase alpha inhibition by aphidicolin induces gaps and breaks at common fragile sites in human chromosomes. Human Genetics. 1984;67(2):136–42. DOI: 10.1007/bf00272988.

[75] Arlt MF, Glover TW. Inhibition of topoisomerase I prevents chromosome breakage at common fragile sites. DNA repair. 2010;9(6):678–89. DOI: 10.1016/j.dnarep.2010.03.005.

[76] Shiraishi T, Druck T, Mimori K, Flomenberg J, Berk L, Alder H, Miller W, Huebner K, Croce CM. Sequence conservation at human and mouse orthologous common fragile regions, FRA3B/FHIT and Fra14A2/Fhit. Proceedings of the National Academy of Sciences of the United States of America. 2001;98(10):5722–7. DOI: 10.1073/pnas.091095898.

[77] Krummel KA, Denison SR, Calhoun E, Phillips LA, Smith DI. The common fragile site FRA16D and its associated gene WWOX are highly conserved in the mouse at Fra8E1. Genes, chromosomes & cancer. 2002;34(2):154–67. DOI: 10.1002/gcc.10047.

[78] Schmid M, Ott G, Haaf T, Scheres JM. Evolutionary conservation of fragile sites induced by 5-azacytidine and 5-azadeoxycytidine in man, gorilla, and chimpanzee. Human Genetics. 1985;71(4):342–50. DOI: 10.1007/bf00388461.

[79] Kang S, Ohshima K, Shimizu M, Amirhaeri S, Wells RD. Pausing of DNA Synthesis in Vitro at Specific Loci in CTG and CGG Triplet Repeats from Human Hereditary Disease Genes. Journal of Biological Chemistry. 1995;270(45):27014–27021. DOI: 10.1074/jbc.270.45.27014.

[80] Zlotorynski E, Rahat A, Skaug J, Ben-Porat N, Ozeri E, Hershberg R, Levi A, Scherer SW, Margalit H, Kerem B. Molecular basis for expression of common and rare fragile sites. Molecular and Cellular Biology. 2003;23(20):7143–51. DOI: 10.1128/mcb.23.20.7143-7151.2003.

[81] Luck G, Zimmer C, Reinert KE, Arcamone F. Specific interactions of distamycin A and its analogs with (A-T) rich and (G-C) rich duplex regions of DNA and deoxypolynucleotides. Nucleic Acids Research. 1977;4(8):2655–70. DOI: 10.1093/nar/4.8.2655.

[82] Balakumaran BS, Freudenreich CH, Zakian VA. CGG/CCG repeats exhibit orientation-dependent instability and orientation-independent fragility in Saccharomyces cerevisiae. Human Molecular Genetics. 2000;9(1):93–100. DOI: 10.1093/hmg/9.1.93.

[83] Yu S, Mangelsdorf M, Hewett D, Hobson L, Baker E, Eyre HJ, Lapsys N, Le Paslier D, Doggett NA, Sutherland GR, Richards RI. Human chromosomal fragile site FRA16B is an amplified AT-rich minisatellite repeat. Cell. 1997;88(3):367–74. DOI: 10.1016/S0092-8674(00)81875-9.

[84] Zhang H, Freudenreich CH. An AT-Rich Sequence in Human Common Fragile Site FRA16D Causes Fork Stalling and Chromosome Breakage in S. cerevisiae. Molecular Cell. 2007;27(3):367–379. DOI: 10.1016/j.molcel.2007.06.012.

[85] Aguilera A, Gómez-González B. Genome instability: A mechanistic view of its causes and consequences. Nature reviews. Genetics. 2008;9(3):204–17. DOI: 10.1038/nrg2268.

[86] Casper AM, Nghiem P, Arlt MF, Glover TW. ATR regulates fragile site stability. Cell. 2002;111:779–789. DOI: http://dx.doi.org/10.1016/S0092-8674(02)01113-3.

[87] Gorgoulis VG, Vassiliou LV, Karakaidos P, Zacharatos P, Kotsinas A, Liloglou T, Venere M, Ditullio RA Jr, Kastrinakis NG, Levy B, Kletsas D, Yoneta A, Herlyn M, Kittas C, Halazonetis TD. Activation of the DNA damage checkpoint and genomic instability in human precancerous lesions. Nature. 2005;434:907–913. DOI: 10.1038/nature03485.

[88] Bartkova J, Horejsí Z, Koed K, Krämer A, Tort F, Zieger K, Guldberg P, Sehested M, Nesland JM, Lukas C, Ørntoft T, Lukas J, Bartek J. DNA damage response as a candidate anti-cancer barrier in early human tumorigenesis. Nature. 2005;434:864–870.

[89] Coquelle A, Pipiras E, Toledo F, Buttin G, Debatisse M. Expression of fragile sites triggers intrachromosomal mammalian gene amplification and sets boundaries to early amplicons. Cell. 1997;89:215–225. DOI: http://dx.doi.org/10.1016/S0092-8674(00)80201-9.

[90] Kuo MT, Vyas RC, Jiang LX, Hittelman WN. Chromosome breakage at a major fragile site associated with P-glycoprotein gene amplification in multidrugresistant CHO cells. Mol. Cell. Biol. 1994;14:5202–5211. DOI: 10.1128/MCB.14.8.5202.

[91] Miller CT, Lin L, Casper AM, Lim J, Thomas DG, Orringer MB, Chang AC, Chambers AF, Giordano TJ, Glover TW, Beer DG. Genomic amplification of MET with boundaries within fragile site FRA7G and upregulation of MET pathways in esophageal adenocarcinoma. Oncogene. 2006;25:409–418. DOI: 10.1038/sj.onc.1209057.

[92] Wang ND, Testa JR, Smith DI. Determination of the specificity of aphidicolin-induced breakage of the human 3pl4.2 fragile site. Genomics. 1993;17:341–347. DOI: 10.1006/geno.1993.1330.

[93] Göker E, Waltham M, Kheradpour A, Trippett T, Mazumdar M, Elisseyeff Y, Schnieders B, Steinherz P, Tan C, Berman E. Amplification of the dihydrofolate reductase gene is a mechanism of acquired resistance to methotrexate in patients with acute lymphoblastic leukemia and is correlated with p53 gene mutations. Blood. 1995;86(2):677–84.

[94] Al-Kuraya K, Schraml P, Torhorst J, Tapia C, Zaharieva B, Novotny H, Spichtin H, Maurer R, Mirlacher M, Köchli O, Zuber M, Dieterich H, Mross F, Wilber K, Simon R, Sauter G. Prognostic relevance of gene amplifications and coamplifications in breast cancer. Cancer Res. 2004;64:8534–8540. DOI: 10.1158/0008-5472.CAN-04-1945.

[95] Blegen H, Will JS, Ghadimi BM, Nash HP, Zetterberg A, Auer G, Ried T. DNA amplifications and aneuploidy, high proliferative activity and impaired cell cycle control characterize breast carcinomas with poor prognosis. Anal. Cell. Pathol. 2003;25:103–114.

[96] Schwab M, Alitalo K, Klempnauer KH, Varmus HE, Bishop JM, Gilbert F, Brodeur G, Goldstein M, Trent J. Amplified DNA with limited homology to myc cellular oncogene is shared by human neuroblastoma cell lines and a neuroblastoma tumour. Nature. 1983;305:245–8.

[97] Savelyeva L, Schwab M. Amplification of oncogenes revisited: From expression profiling to clinical application. Cancer Lett. 2001;167:115–123. DOI: http://dx.doi.org/10.1016/S0304-3835(01)00472-4.

[98] Várkondi E, Gyory F, Nagy A, Kiss I, Ember I, Kozma L. Oncogene amplification and overexpression of oncoproteins in thyroid papillary cancer. In Vivo. 2005;19(2):465–70.

[99] Croce CM. Oncogenes and Cancer. N Engl J Med. 2008;358:502–11. DOI: 10.1056/NEJMra072367.

[100] Yu W, Imoto I, Inoue J, Onda M, Emi M, Inazawa J. A novel amplification target, DUSP26, promotes anaplastic thyroid cancer cell growth by inhibiting p38 MAPK activity. Oncogene. 2007;26(8):1178–87. DOI: 10.1038/sj.onc.1209899.

[101] Anzick SL, Kononen J, Walker RL, Azorsa DO, Tanner MM, Guan XY, Sauter G, Kallioniemi OP, Trent JM, Meltzer PS. AIB1, a steroid receptor coactivator amplified in breast and ovarian cancer. Science. 1997;277:965–968. DOI: 10.1126/science.277.5328.965.

[102] Lahusen T, Henke RT, Kagan BL, Wellstein A, Riegel AT. The role and regulation of the nuclear receptor co-activator AIB1 in breast cancer. Breast Cancer Res Treat. 2009;116:225–237. DOI: 10.1007/s10549-009-0405-2.

[103] Ory V, Tassi E, Cavalli LR, Sharif GM, Saenz F, Baker T, Schmidt MO, Mueller SC, Furth PA, Wellstein A, Riegel AT. The nuclear coactivator amplified in breast cancer 1 maintains tumor-initiating cells during development of ductal carcinoma in situ. Oncogene. 2014;33(23):3033–42. DOI: 10.1038/onc.2013.263.

[104] York B, O'Malley BW. Steroid receptor coactivator (SRC) family: Masters of systems biology. J Biol Chem. 2010;285:38743–38750. DOI: 10.1074/jbc.R110.193367.

[105] Ma YY, Wei SJ, Lin YC, Lung JC, Chang TC, Whang-Peng J, Liu JM, Yang DM, Yang WK, Shen CY. PIK3CA as an oncogene in cervical cancer. Oncogene. 2000;19(23):2739–44.

[106] Chen S, Auletta T, Dovirak O, Hutter C, Kuntz K, El-ftesi S, Kendall J, Han H, Von Hoff DD, Ashfaq R, Maitra A, Iacobuzio-Donahue CA, Hruban RH, Lucito R. Copy number alterations in pancreatic cancer identify recurrent PAK4 amplification. Cancer Biol Ther. 2008;7(11):1793–802. DOI: 10.4161/cbt.7.11.6840.

[107] Pan JS, Cai JY, Xie CX, Zhou F, Zhang ZP, Dong J, Xu HZ, Shi HX, Ren JL. Interacting with HBsAg compromises resistance of jumping translocation breakpoint protein to ultraviolet radiation-induced apoptosis in 293FT cells. Cancer Lett. 2009;285:151–6. DOI: 10.1016/j.canlet.2009.05.009.

[108] Huebner K, Kastury K, Druck T, Salcini AE, Lanfrancone L, Pelicci G, Lowenstein E, Li W, Park SH, Cannizzaro L. Chromosome locations of genes encoding human signal transduction adapter proteins, Nck (NCK), Shc (SHC1), and Grb2 (GRB2). Genomics. 1994;22:281–7. DOI: 10.1006/geno.1994.1385.

[109] Kraut-Cohen J, Muller WJ, Elson A. Protein-tyrosine phosphatase epsilon regulates Shc signaling in a kinase-specific manner: Increasing coherence in tyrosine phosphatase signaling. J Biol Chem. 2008;283:4612–21. DOI: 10.1074/jbc.M708822200.

[110] Shen DY, Fang ZX, You P, Liu PG, Wang F, Huang CL, Yao XB, Chen ZX, Zhang ZY. Clinical significance and expression of cyclin kinase subunits 1 and 2 in hepatocellular carcinoma. Liver Int. 2009;30:19–25. DOI: 10.1111/j.1478-3231.2009.02106.x.

[111] Chen L, Chan TH, Guan XY. Chromosome 1q21 amplification and oncogenes in hepatocellular carcinoma. Acta Pharmacol Sin. 2010;31(9):1165-71. DOI: 10.1038/aps.2010.94.

[112] Zhang S, Liang X, Zheng X, Huang H, Chen X, Wu K, Wang B, Ma S, Glo1 genetic amplification as a potential therapeutic target in hepatocellular carcinoma. Int J Clin Exp Pathol. 2014;7(5):2079–90.

[113] Mariani O, Brennetot C, Coindre JM, Gruel N, Ganem C, Delattre O, Stern MH, Aurias A. JUN oncogene amplification and overexpression block adipocytic differentiation in highly aggressive sarcomas. Cancer Cell. 2007;11(4):361–74. DOI: http://dx.doi.org/10.1016/j.ccr.2007.02.007.

[114] Endo M, Yasui K, Nakajima T, Gen Y, Tsuji K, Dohi O, Zen K, Mitsuyoshi H, Minami M, Itoh Y, Taniwaki M, Tanaka S, Arii S, Okanoue T, Yoshikawa T. Infrequent amplification of JUN in hepatocellular carcinoma. Anticancer Res. 2009;29(12):4989–94.

[115] Eswarakumar VP, Lax I, Schlessinger J. Cellular signaling by fibroblast growth factor receptors. Cytokine Growth Factor Rev. 2005;16:139–49. DOI: http://dx.doi.org/10.1016/j.cytogfr.2005.01.001.

[116] Brooks AN, Kilgour E, Smith PD. Molecular pathways: Fibroblast growth factor signaling: a new therapeutic opportunity in cancer. Clin Cancer Res. 2012;18:1855–62. DOI: 10.1158/1078-0432.CCR-11-0699.

[117] Katoh M, Katoh M. FGF signaling network in the gastrointestinal tract (review). Int J Oncol. 2006;29:163–8. DOI: 10.3892/ijo.29.1.163.

[118] Katoh M. Genetic alterations of FGF receptors: An emerging field in clinical cancer diagnostics and therapeutics. Expert Rev Anticancer Ther. 2010;10:1375–9. DOI: 10.1586/era.10.128.

[119] Grose R, Dickson C. Fibroblast growth factor signaling in tumorigenesis. Cytokine Growth Factor Rev. 2005;16:179–86. DOI: http://dx.doi.org/10.1016/j.cytogfr.2005.01.003.

[120] Xie L, Su X, Zhang L, Yin X, Tang L, Zhang X, Xu Y, Gao Z, Liu K, Zhou M, Gao B, Shen D, Zhang L, Ji J, Gavine PR, Zhang J, Kilgour E, Zhang X, Ji Q. FGFR2 gene amplification in gastric cancer predicts sensitivity to the selective FGFR inhibitor AZD4547. Clin Cancer Res. 2013;19(9):2572–83. DOI: 10.1158/1078-0432.CCR-12-3898.

[121] Mitelman F, Johansson B and Mertens F. The impact of translocations and gene fusions on cancer causation. Nat Rev Cancer. 2007;7:233–245. DOI: 10.1038/nrc2091.

[122] Nambiar M, Kari V and Raghavan SC. Chromosomal translocations in cancer. Biochim Biophys Acta. 2008;1786:139–152. DOI: 10.1016/j.bbcan.2008.07.005.

[123] Fröhling S and Döhner H. Chromosomal abnormalities in cancer. N Engl J Med. 2008;359:722–734. DOI: 10.1056/NEJMra0803109.

[124] Pui CH, Relling MV and Downing JR. Acute lymphoblastic leukemia. N Engl J Med. 2004;350:1535–1548.

[125] Soupir CP, Dal Cin P, Muzikansky A, Kantarjian H, Jones D, Hasserjian RP. Philadelphia chromosome-positive acute myeloid leukemia: A rare aggressive leukemia with clinicopathologic features distinct from chronic myeloid leukemia in myeloid blast crisis. Am J Clin Pathol. 2007;127(4):642–50. DOI: 10.1016/S0140-6736(08)60457-2.

[126] Collins SJ. Retinoic acid receptors, hematopoiesis and leukemogenesis. Curr Opin Hematol. 2008;15:346–351. DOI: 10.1097/MOH.0b013e3283007edf.

[127] Stams WA, den Boer ML, Beverloo HB, Meijerink JP, van Wering ER, Janka-Schaub GE, Pieters R. 2005; Expression levels of TEL, AML1, and the fusion products TEL-AML1 and AML1-TEL versus drug sensitivity and clinical outcome in t(12;21)-positive pediatric acute lymphoblastic leukemia. Clin. Cancer Res. 2005;11(8):2974–80. DOI: 10.1158/1078-0432.CCR-04-1829.

[128] Roix JJ, McQueen PG, Munson PJ, Parada LA and Misteli T. Spatial proximity of translocation-prone gene loci in human lymphomas. Nat Genet. 2011;34:287–291. DOI: 10.1038/ng1177.

[129] Misteli T. The inner life of the genome. Sci Am. 2003;304:66–73.

[130] Osborne CS, Chakalova L, Mitchell JA, Horton A, Wood AL, Bolland DJ, Corcoran AE, Fraser P. *Myc* dynamically and preferentially relocates to a transcription factory occupied by *Igh*. PLoS Biol. 2007;5:e1922007. DOI: 10.1371/journal.pbio.0050192.

[131] Gandhi M, Evdokimova V and Nikiforov YE. Mechanisms of chromosomal rearrangements in solid tumors: The model of papillary thyroid carcinoma. Mol Cell Endocrinol. 2010;321:36–43. DOI: 10.1016/j.mce.2009.09.013.

[132] Merolla F, Pentimalli F, Pacelli R, Vecchio G, Fusco A, Grieco M, Celetti A. Involvement of H4(D10S170) protein in ATM-dependent response to DNA damage. Oncogene. 2007;26:6167–6175. DOI: 10.1038/sj.onc.1210446.

[133] Nikiforov YE. Thyroid carcinoma: Molecular pathways and therapeutic targets. Mod Pathol. 2008;21(2):S37–S43. DOI: 10.1038/modpathol.2008.10.

[134] Ciampi R, Giordano TJ, Wikenheiser-Brokamp K, Koenig RJ, Nikiforov YE. HOOK3-RET: A novel type of RET/PTC rearrangement in papillary thyroid carcinoma. Endocr Relat Cancer. 2007;14:445–452. DOI: 10.1677/ERC-07-0039.

[135] Gandhi M, Medvedovic M, Stringer JR, Nikiforov YE. Interphase chromosome folding determines spatial proximity of genes participating in carcinogenic RET/PTC rearrangements. Oncogene. 2006;25:2360–2366. DOI: 10.1038/sj.onc.1209268.

[136] Sankar S, Lessnick SL. Promiscuous partnerships in Ewing's sarcoma. Cancer Genet. 2011;204:351–365. DOI: 10.1016/j.cancergen.2011.07.008.

[137] Patel M, Simon JM, Iglesia MD, Wu SB, McFadden AW, Lieb JD, Davis IJ. Tumor-specific retargeting of an oncogenic transcription factor chimera results in dysregulation of chromatin and transcription. Genome Res. 2012;22:259–270. DOI: 10.1101/gr.125666.111.

[138] Zelent A, Greaves M, Enver T. Role of the *TEL-AML1* fusion gene in the molecular pathogenesis of childhood acute lymphoblastic leukaemia. Oncogene. 2004;23:4275–4283. DOI: 10.1038/sj.onc.1207672.

[139] Bohlander SK. ETV6: A versatile player in leukemogenesis. Semin Cancer Biol. 2005;15:162–174. DOI: 10.1016/j.semcancer.2005.01.008.

[140] Lin C, Yang L, Tanasa B, Hutt K, Ju BG, Ohgi K, Zhang J, Rose DW, Fu XD, Glass CK, Rosenfeld MG. Nuclear receptor-induced chromosomal proximity and DNA breaks underlie specific translocations in cancer. Cell. 2009;139:1069–1083. DOI: 10.1016/j.cell.2009.11.030.

[141] Li Z, Tognon CE, Godinho FJ, Yasaitis L, Hock H, Herschkowitz JI, Lannon CL, Cho E, Kim SJ, Bronson RT, Perou CM, Sorensen PH, Orkin SH. *ETV6-NTRK3* fusion oncogene initiates breast cancer from committed mammary progenitors via activation of AP1 complex. Cancer Cell. 2007;12:542–558. DOI: http://dx.doi.org/10.1016/j.ccr.2007.11.012.

[142] Seth A, Watson DK. ETS transcription factors and their emerging roles in human cancer. Eur J Cancer. 2005;41:2462–2478.

[143] Gama-Sosa MA, Slagel VA, Trewyn RW, Oxenhandler R, Kuo KC, Gehrke CW, Ehrlich M. The 5-methylcytosine content of DNA from human tumors. Nucleic Acids Res. 1983;11:6883–6894. DOI: 10.1093/nar/11.19.6883.

[144] Ehrlich M. DNA hypomethylation in cancer cells Epigenomics. 2009;1(2):239–259. DOI: 10.2217/epi.09.33.

[145] Alvarez H, Opalinska J, Zhou L, Sohal D, Fazzari MJ, Yu Y, Montagna C, Montgomery EA, Canto M, Dunbar KB, Wang J, Roa JC, Mo Y, Bhagat T, Ramesh KH, Cannizzaro L, Mollenhauer J, Thompson RF, Suzuki M, Meltzer SJ, Melnick A, Greally JM, Maitra A,Verma A. Widespread hypomethylation occurs early and synergizes with gene ampli fi cation during esophageal carcinogenesis. PLoS Genet. 2011;7(3):e1001356. DOI: 10.1371/journal.pgen.1001356.

[146] Sandoval J, Heyn HA, Moran S, Serra-Musach J, Pujana MA, Bibikova M, Esteller M. Validation of a DNA methylation microarray for 450,000 CpG sites in the human genome.Epigenetics. 2011;6(6):692–702. DOI: 10.4161/epi.6.6.16196.

[147] Ruike Y, Imanaka Y, Sato F, Shimizu K, Tsujimoto G. Genome-wide analysis of aberrant methylation in human breast cancer cells using methyl-DNA immunoprecipitation combined with high-throughput sequencing. BMC Genomics. 2010;11:137. DOI: 10.1186/1471-2164-11-137.

[148] Hansen KD, Timp W, Bravo HC, Sabunciyan S, Langmead B, McDonald OG, Wen B, Wu H, Liu Y, Diep D, Briem E, Zhang K, Irizarry RA, Feinberg AP. Increased methylationvariation in epigenetic domains across cancer types. Nat Genet. 2011;43(8):768–775. DOI: 10.1038/ng.865.

[149] Ferguson AT, Vertino PM, Spitzner JR, Baylin SB, Muller MT, Davidson NE. Role of estrogen receptor gene demethylation and DNA methyltransferase. DNA adduct formation in 5-aza-2'deoxycytidine-induced cytotoxicity in human breast cancer cells. J Biol Chem. 1997;272:32260–32266. DOI: 10.1074/jbc.272.51.32260.

[150] Ehrlich M. DNA hypomethylation, cancer, the immunodeficiency, centromeric region instability, facial anomalies syndrome and chromosomal rearrangements. J Nutr. 2002;132:2424S–2429S.

[151] Ehrlich M, Woods CB, Yu MC, Dubeau L, Yang F, Campan M, Weisenberger DJ, Long T, Youn B, Fiala ES, Laird PW. Quantitative analysis of associations between DNA hypermethylation, hypomethylation, and DNMT RNA levels in ovarian tumors. Oncogene. 2006;25:2636–2645. DOI: 10.1038/sj.onc.1209145.

[152] Cash HL, Tao L, Yuan JM, Marsit CJ, Houseman EA, Xiang YB, Gao YT, Nelson HH, Kelsey KT. LINE-1hypomethylation is associated with bladder cancer risk among nonsmoking Chinese. Int J Cancer. 2012;130(5):1151–9. DOI: 10.1002/ijc.26098.

[153] Eden A, Gaudet F, Waghmare A, Jaenisch R. Chromosomal instability and tumors promoted by DNA hypomethylation. Science. 2003;300(5618):455. DOI: 10.1126/science.1083557.

[154] Yamada Y, Jackson-Grusby L, Linhart H, Meissner A, Eden A, Lin H, Jaenisch R. Opposing effects of DNA hypomethylation on intestinal and liver carcinogenesis. Proc NatlAcad Sci USA. 2005;102(38):13580–13585. DOI: 10.1073/pnas.0506612102.

[155] Cadieux B, Ching TT, Vandenberg SR, Costello JF. Genome-wide hypomethylation in human glioblastomas associated with specific copy number alteration, methylenetetrahydrofolatereductase allele status, and increased proliferation. Cancer Res. 2006;66(17):8469–8476. DOI: 10.1158/0008-5472.CAN-06-1547.

[156] Goering W, Ribarska T, Schulz WA. Selective changes of retroelement expression in human prostate cancer. Carcinogenesis. 2011;32(10):1484–92. DOI: 10.1093/carcin/bgr181.

[157] Pulukuri SM, Estes N, Patel J, Rao JS. Demethylation-linked activation of urokinase plasminogen activator is involved in progression of prostate cancer. Cancer Res. 2007;67:930–939. DOI: 10.1158/0008-5472.CAN-06-2892.

[158] Bird A. DNA methylation patterns and epigenetic memory. Genes Dev. 2002;16:6–21. DOI: 10.1101/gad.947102.

[159] Fazzari MJ, Greally JM. Epigenomics: Beyond CpG islands. Nat. Rev.Genet. 2004;5:446–455. DOI: 10.1038/nrg1349.

[160] Tuck-Muller CM, Narayan A, Tsien F, Smeets DF, Sawyer J, Fiala ES, Sohn OS, Ehrlich M. DNA hypomethylation and unusual chromosome instability in cell lines from ICF syndrome patients, Cytogenet. Cell Genet. 2000;89:121–128. DOI: 10.1159/000015590.

[161] Reik W, Dean W, Walter J. Epigenetic reprogramming in mammalian development. Science. 2001;293:1089–1093. DOI: 10.1126/science.1063443.

[162] Avner P, Heard E. X-chromosome inactivation: Counting, choice and initiation. Nat. Rev. Genet. 2001;2:59–67. DOI: 10.1038/35047580.

[163] Pfeifer GP, Rauch TA. DNA methylation patterns in lung carcinomas. Semin Cancer Biol. 2009;19(3):181–187. DOI: 10.1016/j.semcancer.2009.02.00.

[164] Park SY, Yoo EJ, Cho NY, Kim N, Kang GH. Comparison of CpG island hypermethylation and repetitive DNA hypomethylation in premalignant stages of gastric cancer, stratified for Helicobacter pylori infection. J Pathol. 2009;219(4):410–6. DOI: 10.1002/path.2596.

[165] Ehrlich M. Cancer-linked DNA hypomethylation and its relationship to hypermethylation. Curr Top Microbiol Immunol. 2006;310:251–274.

[166] Ehrlich M. DNA methylation in cancer: Too much, but also too little. Oncogene. 2002;21(35):5400–5413. DOI: 10.1038/sj.onc.1205651.

[167] Feber A, Wilson GA, Zhang L, Presneau N, Idowu B, Down TA, Rakyan VK, Noon LA, Lloyd AC, Stupka E, Schiza V, Teschendorff AE, Schroth GP, Flanagan A, Beck S. Comparative methylome analysis of benign and malignant peripheral nerve sheath tumors. Genome Res. 2011;21(4):515–524. DOI: 10.1101/gr.109678.110.

[168] Rodriguez J, Vives L, Jorda M, Morales C, Munoz M, Vendrell E, Peinado MA. Genome-wide tracking of unmethylated DNA Alu repeats in normal and cancer cells. Nucleic Acids Res. 2008;36(3):770–784. DOI: 10.1093/nar/gkm1105.

[169] Wilson AS, Power BE, Molloy PL. DNA hypomethylation and human diseases Biochimica et Biophysica Acta. 2007;1775(1):138–162. DOI: 10.1016/j.bbcan.2006.08.007.

[170] Feinberg AP, Tycko B. The history of cancer epigenetics. Nat. Rev. Cancer. 2004;4:143–153. DOI: 10.1038/nrc1279.

[171] Widschwendter M, Jiang G, Woods C, Muller HM, Fiegl H, Goebel G, Marth C, Holzner EM, Zeimet AG, Laird PW, Ehrlich M. DNA hypomethylation and ovarian cancer biology. Cancer Res. 2004;64(13):4472–4480. DOI: 10.1158/0008-5472.CAN-04-0238.

[172] Ehrlich M, Hopkins N, Jiang G, Dome JS, Yu MS, Woods CB, Tomlinson GE, Chintagumpala M, Champagne M, Diller L, Parham DM, Sawyer J. Satellite hypomethylation in karyotyped Wilms tumors. Cancer Genet Cytogenet. 2003;141:97–105. DOI: http://dx.doi.org/10.1016/S0165-4608(02)00668-4.

[173] Narayan A, Ji W, Zhang X-Y, Marrogi A, Graff JR, Baylin SB, Ehrlich M. Hypomethylation of pericentromeric DNA in breast adenocarcinomas. Int J Cancer. 1998;77:833–838. DOI: 10.1002/(SICI)1097-0215(19980911)77:6<833::AID-IJC6>3.0.CO;2-V.

[174] Qu G, Dubeau L, Narayan A, Yu M, Ehrlich M. Satellite DNA hypomethylation vs. overall genomic hypomethylation in ovarian epithelial tumors of different malignant potential. Mut Res. 1999;423:91–101. DOI: 10.1016/S0027-5107(98)00229-2.

[175] Roman AC, Gonzalez-Rico FJ, Molto E, Hernando H, Neto A, Vicente-Garcia C, Ballestar E, Gomez-Skarmeta JL, Vavrova-Anderson J, White RJ, Montoliu L, Fernandez-Salguero PM. Dioxin receptor and SLUG transcription factors regulate the insulator activity of B1 SINE retrotransposons via an RNA polymerase switch. Genome Res. 2011;21(3):422–432. DOI: 10.1101/gr.111203.110.

[176] Wang J, Lunyak VV, Jordan IK. Genome-wide prediction and analysis of human chromatin boundary elements. Nucleic Acids Res. 2011;40(2):511–29. DOI: 10.1093/nar/gkr750.

[177] Hansen KD, Timp W, Bravo HC, Sabunciyan S, Langmead B, McDonald OG, Wen B, Wu H, Liu Y, Diep D, Briem E, Zhang K, Irizarry RA, Feinberg AP. Increased methylation variation in epigenetic domains across cancer types. Nat Genet. 2011;43(8):768–775. DOI: 10.1038/ng.865.

[178] Irizarry RA, Ladd-Acosta C, Wen B, Wu Z, Montano C, Onyango P, Cui H, Gabo K, Rongione, M, Webster M, Ji H, Potash JB, Sabunciyan S, Feinberg AP. The human colon cancer methylome shows similar hypo- and hypermethylation at conserved tissue-speci fi c CpG island shores. Nat Genet. 2009;41(2):178–186. DOI: 10.1038/ng.298.

[179] Brenet F, Moh M, Funk P, Feierstein E, Viale AJ, Socci ND, Scandura JM. DNA methylation of the fi rst exon is tightly linked to transcriptional silencing. PLoS One. 2011;6(1):e14524. DOI: 10.1371/journal.pone.0014524.

[180] Andrews J, Kennette W, Pilon J, Hodgson A, Tuck AB, Chambers AF, Rodenhiser DI. Multi-platform whole-genome microarray analyses refine the epigenetic signature of breast cancer metastasis with gene expression and copy number. PLoS One. 2010;5(1):e8665. DOI: 10.1371/journal.pone.0008665.

[181] Coolen MW, Stirzaker C, Song JZ, Statham AL, Kassir Z, Moreno CS, Young AN, Varma V, Speed TP, Cowley M, Lacaze P, Kaplan W, Robinson MD, Clark SJ. Consol-

idation of the cancer genome into domains of repressive chromatin by long-range epigenetic silencing (LRES) reduces transcriptional plasticity. Nat Cell Biol. 2010;12(3): 235–246. DOI: 10.1038/ncb2023.

[182] Widschwendter M, Jiang G, Woods C, Muller HM, Fiegl H, Goebel G, Marth C, Holzner EM, Zeimet AG, Laird PW, Ehrlich M. DNA hypomethylation and ovarian cancer biology. Cancer Res. 2004;64(13):4472–4480. DOI: 10.1158/0008-5472.CAN-04-0238.

[183] Dante R, Dante-Paire J, Rigal D, Roizes G. Methylation patterns of long interspersed repeated DNA and alphoid repetitive DNA from human cell lines and tumors. Anticancer Res. 1992;12(2):559–563.

[184] Weisenberger DJ, Campan M, Long TI, Kim M, Woods C, Fiala E, Ehrlich M, Laird PW. Analysis of repetitive element DNA methylation by MethyLight. Nucleic Acids Res. 2005;33(21):6823–6836. DOI: 10.1093/nar/gki987.

[185] Schulz WA, Steinhoff C, Florl AR. Methylation of endogenous human retroelements in health and disease. Curr Top Microbiol Immunol. 2006;310:211–250.

[186] Chan SW, Zilberman D, Xie Z, Johansen LK, Carrington JC, Jacobsen SE. RNA silencing genes control de novo DNA methylation. Science. 2004;303(5662):1336. DOI: DOI: 10.1126/science.1095989.

[187] Qu G (a), Grundy PE, Narayan A, Ehrlich M. Frequent hypomethylation in Wilms tumors of pericentromeric DNA in chromosomes 1 and 16. Cancer Genet Cytogenet. 1999;109:34–39. DOI: http://dx.doi.org/10.1016/S0165-4608(98)00143-5.

[188] Thoraval D, Asakawa J, Wimmer K, Kuick R, Lamb B, Richardson B, Ambros P, Glover T, Hanash S. Demethylation of repetitive DNA sequences in neuroblastoma. Genes Chromosomes Cancer. 1996;17(4):234–244. DOI: 10.1016/S0027-5107(98)00229-2.

[189] Nagai H, Baba M, Konishi N, Kim YS, Nogami M, Okumura K, Emi M, Matsubara K. Isolation of NotI clusters hypomethylated in HBV-integrated hepatocellular carcinomas by two-dimensional electrophoresis. DNA Res. 1999;6(4):219–225. DOI: 10.1093/dnares/6.4.219.

[190] Itano O, Ueda M, Kikuchi K, Hashimoto O, Hayatsu S, Kawaguchi M, Seki H, Aiura K, Kitajima M. Correlation of postoperative recurrence in hepatocellular carcinoma with demethylation of repetitive sequences. Oncogene. 2002;21(5):789–797. DOI: 10.1038/sj/onc/1205124.

[191] Katargin AN, Pavlova LS, Kisseljov FL, Kisseljova NP. Hypermethylation of genomic 3.3-kb repeats is frequent event in HPV-positive cervical cancer. BMC Med Genomics. 2009;2:30. DOI: 10.1186/1755-8794-2-30.

[192] Szpakowski S, Sun X, Lage JM, Dyer A, Rubinstein J, Kowalski D, Sasaki C, Costa J, Lizardi PM. Loss of epigenetic silencing in tumors preferentially affects primate-speci fi c retroelements. Gene. 2009;48(2):151–167. DOI: 10.1016/j.gene.2009.08.006.

[193] Choi SH, Worswick S, Byun HM, Shear T, Soussa JC, Wolff EM, Douer D, Garcia-Manero, G, Liang G, Yang AS. Changes in DNA methylation of tandem DNA repeats are different from interspersed repeats in cancer. Int J Cancer. 2009;125(3):723–729. DOI: 10.1002/ijc.24384.

[194] Itano O, Ueda M, Kikuchi K, Shimazu M, Kitagawa Y, Aiura K, Kitajima M. A new predictive factor for hepatocellular carcinoma based on two- dimensional electrophoresis of genomic DNA. Oncogene. 2000;19(13):1676–1683.

[195] Grunau C, Sanchez C, Ehrlich M, van der Bruggen P, Hindermann W, Rodriguez C, Krieger S, De Sario A. Frequent DNA hypomethylation in the human juxtacentromeric BAGE loci in cancer. Genes Chrom Cancer. 2005;43(1):11–24. DOI: 10.1002/gcc.20155.

[196] Roman-Gomez J, Jimenez-Velasco A, Agirre X, Castillejo JA, Navarro G, San Jose-Eneriz E, Garate L, Cordeu L, Cervantes F, Prosper F, Heiniger A, Torres A. Repetitive DNA hypomethylation in the advanced phase of chronic myeloid leukemia. Leuk Res. 2008;32(3):487–490. DOI: http://dx.doi.org/10.1016/j.leukres.2007.07.021.

[197] Yegnasubramanian S, Haffner MC, Zhang Y, Gurel B, Cornish TC, Wu Z, Irizarry RA, Morgan J, Hicks J, DeWeese TL, Isaacs WB, Bova GS, De Marzo AM, Nelson WG. DNA hypomethylation arises later in prostate cancer progression than CpG island hypermethylation and contributes to metastatic tumor heterogeneity. Cancer Res. 2008;68(21):8954–8967. DOI: 10.1158/0008-5472.CAN-07-6088.

[198] Horiuchi A, Hayashi T, Kikuchi N, Hayashi A, Fuseya C, Shiozawa T, Konishi I. Hypoxia upregulates ovarian cancer invasiveness via the binding of HIF-1alpha to a hypoxia-induced, methylation-free hypoxia response element of S100A4 gene. Int J Cancer. 2012;131:1755–1767. DOI: 10.1002/ijc.27448.

[199] Irizarry RA, Ladd-Acosta C, Wen B, Wu Z, Montano C, Onyango P, Cui H, Gabo K, Rongione M, Webster M, Ji H, Potash JB, Sabunciyan S, Feinberg AP.The human colon cancer methylome shows similar hypo- and hypermethylation at conserved tissue-specific CpG island shores. Nat Genet. 2009;41:178–186. DOI: 10.1038/ng.298.

[200] Smale ST. Pioneer factors in embryonic stem cells and differentiation. Curr Opin Genet Dev. 2010;20(5):519–526. DOI: 10.1016/j.gde.2010.06.010.

[201] Serandour AA, Avner S, Percevault F, Demay F, Bizot M, Lucchetti-Miganeh C, Barloy-Hubler F, Brown M, Lupien M, Metivier R, Salbert G, Eeckhoute J. Epigenetic switch involved in activation of pioneer factor FOXA1-dependent enhancers. Genome Res. 2011;21(4):555–565. DOI: 10.1101/gr.111534.110.

[202] Taube JH, Allton K, Duncan SA, Shen L, Barton MC. Foxa1 functions as a pioneer transcription factor at transposable elements to activate Afp during differentiation of

embryonic stem cells. J Biol Chem. 2010;285(21):16135–16144. DOI: 10.1074/jbc.M109.088096.

[203] Magnani L, Eeckhoute J, Lupien M. Pioneer factors: Directing transcriptional regulators within the chromatin environment. Trends Genet. 2011;27(11):465–74. DOI: 10.1016/j.tig.2011.07.002.

[204] Hatada I, Namihira M, Morita S, Kimura M, Horii T, Nakashima K. Astrocyte-specific genes are generally demethylated in neural precursor cells prior to astrocytic differentiation. PLoS One. 2008;3(9):e3189. DOI: 10.1371/journal.pone.0003189.

[205] Son KS, Kang HS, Kim SJ, Jung SY, Min SY, Lee SY, Kim SW, Kwon Y, Lee KS, Shin KH, Ro J. Hypomethylation of the interleukin-10 gene in breast cancer tissues. Breast. 2010;19:484–488. DOI: 10.1016/j.breast.2010.05.011.

[206] Wang Z, Zhang J, Zhang Y, Lim SH. SPAN-Xb expression in myeloma cells is dependent on promoter hypomethylation and can be upregulated pharmacologically. Int J Cancer. 2006;118:1436–1444. DOI: 10.1002/ijc.21499.

[207] Noushmehr H, Weisenberger DJ, Diefes K, Phillips HS, Pujara K, Berman BP, Pan F, Pelloski CE, Sulman EP, Bhat KP, Verhaak RG, Hoadley KA, Hayes DN, Perou CM, Schmidt HK, Ding L, Wilson RK, Van Den Berg D, Shen H, Bengtsson H, Neuvial P, Cope LM, Buckley J, Herman JG, Baylin SB, Laird PW, Aldape K; Cancer Genome Atlas Research Network. Identification of a CpG island methylator phenotype that defines a distinct subgroup of glioma. Cancer Cell. 2010;17:510–522. DOI: 10.1016/j.ccr.2010.03.017.

[208] Hoffmann MJ, Schulz WA. Causes and consequences of DNA hypomethylation in human cancer. Biochem Cell Biol. 2005;83:296–321. DOI: 10.1139/o05-036.

[209] Eckhardt F, Lewin J, Cortese R, Rakyan VK, Attwood J, Burger M, Burton J, Cox TV, Davies R, Down TA, Hae fl iger C, Horton R, Howe K, Jackson DK, Kunde J, Koenig C, Liddle J, Niblett D, Otto T, Pettett R, Seemann S, Thompson C, West T, Rogers J, Olek A, Berlin K, Beck S. DNA methylation pro fi ling of human chromosomes 6, 20 and 22. Nat Genet. 2006;38(12):1378–1385. DOI: 10.1038/ng1909.

[210] Baba Y, Nosho K, Shima K, Huttenhower C, Tanaka N, Hazra A, Giovannucci EL, Fuchs CS, Ogino S. Hypomethylation of the IGF2 DMR in colorectal tumors, detected by bisulfite pyrosequencing, is associated with poor prognosis. Gastroenterology. 2010;139(6):1855–1864. DOI: 10.1053/j.gastro.2010.07.050.

[211] Ball MP, Li JB, Gao Y, Lee JH, LeProust EM, Park IH, Xie B, Daley GQ, Church GM. Targeted and genome-scale strategies reveal gene-body methylation signatures in human cells. Nat Biotechnol. 2009;27(4):361–368. DOI: 10.1038/nbt.1533.

[212] Wu H, Coskun V, Tao J, Xie W, Ge W, Yoshikawa K, Li E, Zhang Y, Sun YE. Dnmt3a-dependent nonpromoter DNA methylation facilitates transcription of neurogenic genes. Science. 2010;329(5990):444–448. DOI: 10.1126/science.

[213] Lister R, Pelizzola M, Dowen RH, Hawkins RD, Hon G, Tonti-Filippini J, Nery JR, Lee L, Ye Z, Ngo QM, Edsall L, Antosiewicz-Bourget J, Stewart R, Ruotti V, Millar AH, Thomson JA, Ren B, Ecker JR. Human DNA methylomes at base resolution show widespread epigenomic differences. Nature. 2009;462(7271):315–322. DOI: 10.1038/nature08514.

[214] De Bustos C, Ramos E, Young JM, Tran RK, Menzel U, Langford CF, Eichler EE, Hsu L, Henikoff S, Dumanski JP, Trask BJ. Tissue-speci fi c variation in DNA methylation levels along human chromosome 1. Epigenetics Chromatin. 2009;2(1):7. DOI: 10.1186/1756-8935-2-7.

[215] Ke XS, Qu Y, Cheng Y, Li WC, Rotter V, Oyan AM, Kalland KH. Global pro fi ling of histone and DNA methylation reveals epigenetic-based regulation of gene expression during epithelial to mesenchymal transition in prostate cells. BMC Genomics. 2010;11:669. DOI: 10.1186/1471-2164-11-669.

[216] Cheng X, Blumenthal RM. Coordinated chromatin control: Structural and functional linkage of DNA and histone methylation. Biochemistry. 2010;49(14):2999–3008. DOI: 10.1021/bi100213t.

[217] Stengel S, Fiebig U, Kurth R, Denner J. Regulation of human endogenous retrovirus-K expression in melanomas by CpG methylation. Genes Chromosomes Cancer. 2010;49(5):401–411. DOI: 10.1002/gcc.20751.

[218] Appanah R, Dickerson DR, Goyal P, Groudine M, Lorincz MC. An unmethylated 3′ promoter-proximal region is required for ef fi cient transcription initiation. PLoS Genet. 2007;3(2):e27. DOI: 10.1371/journal.pgen.0030027.

[219] Chodavarapu RK, Feng S, Bernatavichute YV, Chen PY, Stroud H, Yu Y, Hetzel JA, Kuo F, Kim J, Cokus SJ, Casero D, Bernal M, Huijser P, Clark AT, Kramer U, Merchant SS, Zhang X, Jacobsen SE, Pellegrini M. Relationship between nucleosome positioning and DNA methylation. Nature. 2010;466(7304):388–392. DOI: 10.1038/nature09147.

[220] Maunakea AK, Nagarajan RP, Bilenky M, Ballinger TJ, D'Souza C, Fouse SD, Johnson BE, Hong C, Nielsen C, Zhao Y, Turecki G, Delaney A, Varhol R, Thiessen N, Shchors K, Heine VM, Rowitch DH, Xing X, Fiore C, Schillebeeckx M, Jones SJ, Haussler D, Marra MA, Hirst M, Wang T, Costello JF. Conserved role of intragenic DNA methylation in regulating alternative promoters. Nature. 2010;466(7303):253–257. DOI: 10.1038/nature09165.

[221] Hodges E, Smith AD, Kendall J, Xuan Z, Ravi K, Rooks M, Zhang MQ, Ye K, Bhattacharjee A, Brizuela L, McCombie WR, Wigler M, Hannon GJ, Hicks JB. High definition profiling of mammalian DNA methylation by array capture and single molecule bisulfite sequencing. Genome Res. 2009;19(9):1593–1605. DOI: 10.1101/gr.095190.109.

[222] Luco RF, Allo M, Schor IE, Kornblihtt AR, Misteli. Epigenetics in alternative pre-mRNA splicing. Cell. 2011;144(1):16–26. DOI: 10.1016/j.cell.2010.11.056.

[223] Laurent L, Wong E, Li G, Huynh T, Tsirigos A, Ong CT, Low HM, Kin Sung KW, Rigoutsos I, Loring J, Wei CL. Dynamic changes in the human methylome during differentiation. Genome Res. 2010;20(3):320–331. DOI: 10.1101/gr.101907.109.

[224] Yegnasubramanian S, Wu Z, Haffner MC, Esopi D, Aryee MJ, Badrinath R, He TL, Morgan JD, Carvalho B, Zheng Q, De Marzo AM, Irizarry RA, Nelson WG. Chromosome wide mapping of DNA methylation patterns in normal and malignant prostate cells reveals pervasive methylation of gene-associated and conserved intergenic sequences. BMC Genomics. 2011;12:313. DOI: 10.1186/1471-2164-12-313.

[225] Nagai H, Kim YS, Yasuda T, Ohmachi Y, Yokouchi H, Monden M, Emi M, Konishi N, Nogami M, Okumura K, Matsubara K. A novel sperm-speci fi c hypomethylation sequence is a demethylation hotspot in human hepatocellular carcinomas. Gene. 1999;237(1):15–20. DOI: 10.1016/S0378-1119(99)00322-4.

[226] Faam B, Ghaffari MA, Ghadiri A, Azizi F. Epigenetic modifications in human thyroid cancer. Biomed Rep. 2015;3(1):3-8. DOI: 10.3892/br.2014.375.

[227] Shen X, He Z, Li H, Yao C, Zhang Y, He L, Li S, Huang J, Guo Z. Distinct functional patterns of gene promoter hypomethylation and hypermethylation in cancer genomes. PLoS One. 2012;7(9):e44822. DOI: 10.1371/journal.pone.0044822.

[228] Nishigaki M, Aoyagi K, Danjoh I, Fukaya M, Yanagihara K, Sakamoto H, Yoshida T, Sasaki H. Discovery of aberrant expression of R-RAS by cancer-linked DNA hypomethylation in gastric cancer using microarrays, Cancer Res. 2005;65:2115–2124. DOI: 10.1158/0008-5472.CAN-04-3340.

[229] Paredes J, Albergaria A, Oliveira JT, Jerónimo C, Milanezi F, Schmitt FC. P-cadherin overexpression is an indicator of clinical outcome in invasive breast carcinomas and is associated with CDH3 promoter hypomethylation. Clin. Cancer Res. 2005;11:5869–5877. DOI: 10.1158/1078-0432.CCR-05-0059.

[230] Oshimo Y, Nakayama H, Ito R, Kitadai Y, Yoshida K, Chayama K, Yasui W. Promoter methylation of cyclin D2 gene in gastric carcinoma, Int. J. Oncol. 2003;23:1663–1670. DOI: 10.3892/ijo.23.6.1663.

[231] Liu H, Liu W, Wu Y, Zhou Y, Xue R, Luo C, Wang L, Zhao W, Jiang JD, Liu J. Loss of epigenetic control of synuclein-gamma gene as a molecular indicator of metastasis in a wide range of human cancers, Cancer Res. 2005;65:7635–7643. DOI: 10.1158/0008-5472.CAN-05-1089.

[232] Bettstetter M, Woenckhaus M, Wild PJ, Rümmele P, Blaszyk H, Hartmann A, Hofstädter F, Dietmaier W. Elevated nuclear maspin expression is associated with microsatellite instability and high tumour grade in colorectal cancer, J. Pathol. 2005;205:606–614. DOI: 10.1002/path.1732.

[233] Holm TM, Jackson-Grusby L, Brambrink T, Yamada Y, Rideout WM 3rd, Jaenisch R. Global loss of imprinting leads to widespread tumorigenesis in adult mice. Cancer Cell. 2005;8:275–285. DOI: http://dx.doi.org/10.1016/j.ccr.2005.09.007.

[234] Pogribny IP, Beland FA. DNA hypomethylation in the origin and pathogenesis of human diseases. Cell Mol Life Sci. 2009;66:2249–2261. DOI: 10.1007/s00018-009-0015-5.

[235] Tycko, B. Genomic imprinting and human neoplasia. In: Ehrlich, M., editor. DNA and Alterations in Cancer: Genetic and Epigenetic Alterations. Eaton Publishing; MA, USA: 2000. p. 333-349.

[236] Søes S, Daugaard IL, Sørensen BS, Carus A, Mattheisen M, Alsner J, Overgaard J, Hager H, Hansen LL, Kristensen LS. Hypomethylation and increased expression of the putative oncogene ELMO3 are associated with lung cancer development and metastases formation. Oncoscience. 2014;1(5):367–74. eCollection 2014.

[237] Wang Q, Williamson M, Bott S, Brookman-Amissah N, Freeman A, Nariculam J, Hubank MJ, Ahmed A, Masters JR. Hypomethylation of WNT5A, CRIP1 and S100P in prostate cancer. Oncogene. 2007;4;26(45):6560–5. DOI: 10.1038/sj.onc.1210472.

[238] Ota A, Tagawa H, Karnan S, Tsuzuki S, Karpas A, Kira S, Yoshida Y, Seto M. Identification and characterization of a novel gene, C13orf25, as a target for 13q31-q32 amplification in malignant lymphoma. Cancer Res. 2004;64(9):3087–95. DOI: 10.1158/0008-5472.CAN-03-3773.

[239] Tagawa H, Seto M. A microRNA cluster as a target of genomic amplification in malignant lymphoma.Leukemia. 2005;19(11):2013–6. DOI: 10.1038/sj.leu.2403942.

[240] Hayashita Y, Osada H, Tatematsu Y, Yamada H, Yanagisawa K, Tomida S, Yatabe Y, Kawahara K, Sekido Y, Takahashi T. A polycistronic microRNA cluster, miR-17-92, is overexpressed in human lung cancers and enhances cell proliferation. Cancer Res. 2005;65(21):9628–32. DOI: 10.1158/0008-5472.CAN-05-2352.

[241] Wang CL, Wang BB, Bartha G, Li L, Channa N, Klinger M, Killeen N, Wabl M. Activation of an oncogenic microRNA cistron by provirus integration.Proc Natl Acad Sci U S A. 2006;103(49):18680–4. DOI: 10.1073/pnas.0609030103.

[242] Woods K, Thomson JM, Hammond SM. Direct regulation of an oncogenic microRNA cluster by E2F transcription factors. J Biol Chem. 2007;282(4):2130–4. DOI: 10.1074/jbc.C600252200.

[243] Sylvestre Y, De Guire V, Querido E, Mukhopadhyay UK, Bourdeau V, Major F, Ferbeyre G, Chartrand P. An E2F/miR-20a autoregulatory feedback loop. J Biol Chem. 2007;282(4):2135–43. DOI: 10.1074/jbc.M608939200.

[244] Fang L, Deng Z, Shatseva T, Yang J, Peng C, Du WW, Yee AJ, Ang LC, He C, Shan SW, Yang BB. MicroRNA miR-93 promotes tumor growth and angiogenesis by targeting integrin-beta8. Oncogene. 2011;30:806–821. DOI: 10.1038/onc.2010.465.

[245] Ivanovska I, Ball AS, Diaz RL, Magnus JF, Kibukawa M, Schelter JM, Kobayashi SV, Lim L, Burchard J, Jackson AL, Linsley PS, Cleary MA. MicroRNAs in the miR-106b family regulate p21/CDKN1A and promote cell cycle progression. Mol Cell Biol. 2008;28:2167–2174. DOI: 10.1128/MCB.01977-07.

[246] Poliseno L, Salmena L, Riccardi L, Fornari A, Song MS, Hobbs RM, Sportoletti P, Varmeh S, Egia A, Fedele G, Rameh L, Loda M, Pandolfi PP. Identification of the miR-106b~25 microRNA cluster as a proto-oncogenic PTEN-targeting intron that cooperates with its host gene MCM7 in transformation. Sci Signal. 2010;3(117):ra29. DOI: 10.1126/scisignal.2000594.

[247] Petrocca F, Visone R, Onelli MR, Shah MH, Nicoloso MS, de Martino I, Iliopoulos D, Pilozzi E, Liu CG, Negrini M, Cavazzini L, Volinia S, Alder H, Ruco LP, Baldassarre G, Croce CM, Vecchione A. E2F1-regulated microRNAs impair TGF[beta]-dependent cell-cycle arrest and apoptosis in gastric cancer. Cancer Cell. 2008;13:272–286. DOI: 10.1016/j.ccr.2008.02.013.

[248] Smith AL, Iwanaga R, Drasin DJ, Micalizzi DS, Vartuli RL, Tan AC, Ford HL. The miR-106b-25 cluster targets Smad7, activates TGF-beta signaling, and induces EMT and tumor initiating cell characteristics downstream of Six1 in human breast cancer. Oncogene. 2012;31:5162–5171. DOI: 10.1038/onc.2012.11.

[249] Zhou Y, Hu Y, Yang M, Jat P, Li K, Lombardo Y, Xiong D, Coombes RC, Raguz S, Yagüe E. The miR-106b~25 cluster promotes bypass of doxorubicin-induced senescence and increase in motility and invasion by targeting the E-cadherin transcriptional activator EP300. Cell Death Differ. 2014;21(3):462–74. DOI: 10.1038/cdd.2013.167.

[250] Volinia S, Calin GA, Liu CG, Ambs S, Cimmino A, Petrocca F, Visone R, Iorio M, Roldo C, Ferracin M, Prueitt RL, Yanaihara N, Lanza G, Scarpa A, Vecchione A, Negrini M, Harris CC, Croce CM. A microRNA expression signature of human solid tumors defines cancer gene targets. Proc Natl Acad Sci U S A. 2006;103:2257–61. DOI: 10.1073/pnas.0510565103.

[251] Yu J, Wang F, Yang GH, Wang FL, Ma YN, Du ZW, Zhang JW. Human microRNA clusters: Genomic organization and expression profile in leukemia cell lines. Biochem Biophys Res Commun. 2006;349:59–68. DOI: 10.1016/j.bbrc.2006.07.207.

[252] Dylla L, Jedlicka P. Growth-promoting role of the miR-106a~363 cluster in Ewing sarcoma. PLoS One. 2013;8(4):e63032. DOI: 10.1371/journal.pone.0063032.

[253] Fulci V, Chiaretti S, Goldoni M, Azzalin G, Carucci N, Tavolaro S, Castellano L, Magrelli A, Citarella F, Messina M, Maggio R, Peragine N, Santangelo S, Mauro FR, Landgraf P, Tuschl T, Weir DB, Chien M, Russo JJ, Ju J, Sheridan R, Sander C, Zavolan M, Guarini A, Foà R, Macino G. Quantitative technologies establish a novel microRNA profile of chronic lymphocytic leukemia. Blood. 2007;109(11):4944–51. DOI: http://dx.doi.org/10.1182/blood-2006-12-062398.

[254] Eis PS, Tam W, Sun L, Chadburn A, Li Z, Gomez MF, Lund E, Dahlberg JE. Accumulation of miR-155 and BIC RNA in human B cell lymphomas. Proc Natl Acad Sci U S A. 20058;102(10):3627–32. DOI: 10.1073/pnas.0500613102.

[255] Metzler M, Wilda M, Busch K, Viehmann S, Borkhardt A. High expression of precursor microRNA-155/BIC RNA in children with Burkitt lymphoma. Genes Chromosomes Cancer. 2004;39(2):167–9. DOI: 10.1002/gcc.10316.

[256] Iorio MV, Ferracin M, Liu CG, Veronese A, Spizzo R, Sabbioni S, Magri E, Pedriali M, Fabbri M, Campiglio M, Ménard S, Palazzo JP, Rosenberg A, Musiani P, Volinia S, Nenci I, Calin GA, Querzoli P, Negrini M, Croce CM. MicroRNA gene expression deregulation in human breast cancer. Cancer Res. 2005;65(16):7065–70. DOI: 10.1158/0008-5472.CAN-05-1783.

[257] Gironella M, Seux M, Xie MJ, Cano C, Tomasini R, Gommeaux J, Garcia S, Nowak J, Yeung ML, Jeang KT, Chaix A, Fazli L, Motoo Y, Wang Q, Rocchi P, Russo A, Gleave M, Dagorn JC, Iovanna JL, Carrier A, Pébusque MJ, Dusetti NJ. Tumor protein 53-induced nuclear protein 1 expression is repressed by miR-155, and its restoration inhibits pancreatic tumor development. Proc Natl Acad Sci U S A. 2007;104(41):16170–5. DOI: 10.1073/pnas.0703942104.

[258] Krichevsky AM, Gabriely G. miR-21: A small multi-faceted RNA. J Cell Mol Med. 2009;13(1):39–53. DOI: 10.1111/j.1582-4934.2008.00556.

[259] Chan JA, Krichevsky AM, Kosik KS: MicroRNA-21 is an antiapoptotic factor in human glioblastoma cells. Cancer Res. 2005;65:6029–6033. DOI: 10.1158/0008-5472.CAN-05-0137.

[260] Iorio MV, Visone R, Di Leva G, Donati V, Petrocca F, Casalini P, Taccioli C, Volinia S, Liu CG, Alder H, Calin GA, Ménard S, Croce CM. MicroRNA signatures in human ovarian cancer. Cancer Res. 2007;67(18):8699–707. DOI: 10.1158/0008-5472.

[261] Lui WO, Pourmand N, Patterson BK, Fire A. Patterns of known and novel small RNAs in human cervical cancer. Cancer Res.2007;67(13):6031–43. DOI: 10.1158/0008-5472.

[262] Hu Y, Correa AM, Hoque A, Guan B, Ye F, Huang J, Swisher SG, Wu TT, Ajani JA, Xu XC. Prognostic significance of differentially expressed miRNAs in esophageal cancer". Int. J. Cancer. 2011;128(1):132–43. DOI: 10.1002/ijc.25330.

[263] Tetzlaff MT, Liu A, Xu X, Master SR, Baldwin DA, Tobias JW, Livolsi VA, Baloch ZW. Differential expression of miRNAs in papillary thyroid carcinoma compared to multinodular goiter using formalin fixed paraffin embedded tissues. Endocr. Pathol. 2007;18(3):163–73. DOI: 10.1007/s12022-007-0023-7.

[264] Asangani IA, Rasheed SA, Nikolova DA, Leupold JH, Colburn NH, Post S, Allgayer H. MicroRNA-21 (miR-21) post-transcriptionally downregulates tumor suppressor

Pdcd4 and stimulates invasion, intravasation and metastasis in colorectal cancer. Oncogene. 2008;27(15):2128–36. DOI: 10.1038/sj.onc.1210856.

[265] Zhu S, Wu H, Wu G, Nie D, Sheng S, Mo YY. MicroRNA-21 targets tumor suppressor genes in invasion and metastasis. Cell Res. 2008;18:350–359. DOI: 10.1038/cr.2008.24.

[266] Cheng AM, Byrom MW, Shelton J, Ford LP. Antisense inhibition of human miRNAs and indications for an involvement of miRNA in cell growth and apoptosis. Nucleic Acids Res. 2005;33(4):1290–7. DOI: 10.1093/nar/gki200.

[267] Papagiannakopoulos T, Shapiro A, Kosik KS. MicroRNA-21 targets a network of key tumor-suppressive pathways in glioblastoma cells. Cancer Res. 2008;68(19):8164–72. DOI: 10.1158/0008-5472.

[268] Gabriely G, Wurdinger T, Kesari S, Esau CC, Burchard J, Linsley PS, Krichevsky AM. MicroRNA 21 promotes glioma invasion by targeting matrix metalloproteinase regulators. 2. Mol Cell Biol. 2008;28(17):5369–80. DOI: 10.1128/MCB.00479-08.

[269] Mandal CC, Ghosh-Choudhury T, Dey N, Choudhury GG, Ghosh-Choudhury N. miR-21 is targeted by omega-3 polyunsaturated fatty acid to regulate breast tumor CSF-1 expression. Carcinogenesis. 2012;33(10):1897–908. DOI: 10.1093/carcin/bgs198.

[270] Wang ZX, Lu BB, Wang H, Cheng ZX, Yin YM. MicroRNA-21 modulates chemosensitivity of breast cancer cells to doxorubicin by targeting PTEN. Arch Med Res. 2011;42(4):281–90. DOI: 10.1016/j.arcmed.2011.06.008.

[271] Yan LX, Wu QN, Zhang Y, Li YY, Liao DZ, Hou JH, Fu J, Zeng MS, Yun JP, Wu QL, Zeng YX, Shao JY. Knockdown of miR-21 in human breast cancer cell lines inhibits proliferation, in vitro migration and in vivo tumor growth. Breast Cancer Res. 2011;13(1):R2. DOI: 10.1186/bcr2803.

[272] Wickramasinghe NS, Manavalan TT, Dougherty SM, Riggs KA, Li Y, Klinge CM. Estradiol downregulates miR-21 expression and increases miR-21 target gene expression in MCF-7 breast cancer cells. Nucleic Acids Res. 2009;37(8):2584–95. DOI: 10.1093/nar/gkp117.

[273] Yao T, Lin Z. MiR-21 is involved in cervical squamous cell tumorigenesis and regulates CCL20.Biochim Biophys Acta. 2012;1822(2):248–60. DOI: 10.1016/j.bbadis.2011.09.018.

[274] Yao Q, Xu H, Zhang QQ, Zhou H, Qu LH. MicroRNA-21 promotes cell proliferation and down-regulates the expression of programmed cell death 4 (PDCD4) in HeLa cervical carcinoma cells. Biochem Biophys Res Commun. 2009;388(3):539–42. DOI: 10.1016/j.bbrc.2009.08.044.

[275] Coppola V, Musumeci M, Patrizii M, Cannistraci A, Addario A, Maugeri-Saccà M, Biffoni M, Francescangeli F, Cordenonsi M, Piccolo S, Memeo L, Pagliuca A, Muto G, Zeuner A, De Maria R, Bonci D. BTG2 loss and miR-21 upregulation contribute to

prostate cell transformation by inducing luminal markers expression and epithelial-mesenchymal transition. Oncogene. 2013;32(14):1843–53. DOI: 10.1038/onc.2012.194.

[276] Liu LZ, Li C, Chen Q, Jing Y, Carpenter R, Jiang Y, Kung HF, Lai L, Jiang BH. MiR-21-induced angiogenesis through AKT and ERK activation and HIF-1α expression. PLoS One. 2011;6(4):e19139. DOI: 10.1371/journal.pone.0019139.

[277] Shi GH, Ye DW, Yao XD, Zhang SL, Dai B, Zhang HL, Shen YJ, Zhu Y, Zhu YP, Xiao WJ, Ma CG. Involvement of microRNA-21 in mediating chemo-resistance to docetaxel in androgen-independent prostate cancer PC3 cells. Acta Pharmacol Sin. 2010;31(7):867–73. DOI: 10.1038/aps.2010.48.

[278] Ribas J, Ni X, Haffner M, Wentzel EA, Salmasi AH, Chowdhury WH, Kudrolli TA, Yegnasubramanian S, Luo J, Rodriguez R, Mendell JT, Lupold SE. miR-21: An androgen receptor-regulated microRNA that promotes hormone-dependent and hormone-independent prostate cancer growth. Cancer Res. 2009;69(18):7165–9. DOI: 10.1158/0008-5472.CAN-09-1448.

[279] Li T, Li D, Sha J, Sun P, Huang Y. MicroRNA-21 directly targets MARCKS and promotes apoptosis resistance and invasion in prostate cancer cells. Biochem Biophys Res Commun. 2009;383(3):280–5. DOI: 10.1016/j.bbrc.2009.03.077.

[280] Hu H, Li Y, Gu J, Zhu X, Dong D, Yao J, Lin C, Fei J. Antisense oligonucleotide against miR-21 inhibits migration and induces apoptosis in leukemic K562 cells. Leuk Lymphoma. 2010;51(4):694–701. DOI: 10.3109/10428191003596835.

[281] Gu J, Zhu X, Li Y, Dong D, Yao J, Lin C, Huang K, Hu H, Fei J. miRNA-21 regulates arsenic-induced anti-leukemia activity in myelogenous cell lines. Med Oncol. 2011;28(1):211–8. DOI: 10.1007/s12032-009-9413-7.

[282] Galardi S, Mercatelli N, Giorda E, Massalini S, Frajese GV, Ciafrè SA, Farace MG. miR-221 and miR-222 expression affects the proliferation potential of human prostate carcinoma cell lines by targeting p27Kip1. J Biol Chem. 2007;282(32):23716–24. DOI: 10.1074/jbc.M701805200.

[283] Stinson S, Lackner MR, Adai AT, Yu N, Kim HJ, O'Brien C, Spoerke J, Jhunjhunwala S, Boyd Z, Januario T, Newman RJ, Yue P, Bourgon R, Modrusan Z, Stern HM, Warming S, de Sauvage FJ, Amler L, Yeh RF, Dornan D. miR-221/222 targeting of trichorhinophalangeal 1 (TRPS1) promotes epithelial-to-mesenchymal transition in breast cancer. Sci Signal. 2011;4(186):pt5. DOI: 10.1126/scisignal.2002258.

[284] Miller TE, Ghoshal K, Ramaswamy B, Roy S, Datta J, Shapiro CL, Jacob S, Majumder S. MicroRNA-221/222 confers tamoxifen resistance in breast cancer by targeting p27Kip1. J Biol Chem. 2008;283(44):29897–903. DOI: 10.1074/jbc.M804612200.

[285] Zhang C, Zhang J, Hao J, Shi Z, Wang Y, Han L, Yu S, You Y, Jiang T, Wang J, Liu M, Pu P, Kang C. High level of miR-221/222 confers increased cell invasion and poor prognosis in glioma. J Transl Med. 2012;10:119. DOI: 10.1186/1479-5876-10-119.

[286] Hao J, Zhang C, Zhang A, Wang K, Jia Z, Wang G, Han L, Kang C, Pu P. miR-221/222 is the regulator of Cx43 expression in human glioblastoma cells. Oncol Rep. 2012;27(5):1504–10. DOI: 10.3892/or.2012.1652.

[287] Visone R, Russo L, Pallante P, De Martino I, Ferraro A, Leone V, Borbone E, Petrocca F, Alder H, Croce CM, Fusco A. MicroRNAs (miR)-221 and miR-222, both overexpressed in human thyroid papillary carcinomas, regulate p27Kip1 protein levels and cell cycle. Endocr Relat Cancer. 2007;14(3):791–8. DOI: 10.1677/ERC-07-0129.

[288] Garofalo M, Di Leva G, Romano G, Nuovo G, Suh SS, Ngankeu A, Taccioli C, Pichiorri F, Alder H, Secchiero P, Gasparini P, Gonelli A, Costinean S, Acunzo M, Condorelli G, Croce CM. miR-221&222 regulate TRAIL resistance and enhance tumorigenicity through PTEN and TIMP3 downregulation. Cancer Cell. 2009;16(6): 498–509. DOI: 10.1016/j.ccr.2009.10.014.

[289] Sandhu SK, Volinia S, Costinean S, Galasso M, Neinast R, Santhanam R, Parthun MR, Perrotti D, Marcucci G, Garzon R, Croce CM. miR-155 targets histone deacetylase 4 (HDAC4) and impairs transcriptional activity of B-cell lymphoma 6 (BCL6) in the Eμ-miR-155 transgenic mouse model. Proc Natl Acad Sci U S A. 2012;109(49):20047–52. DOI: 10.1073/pnas.1213764109.

[290] Huang X, Shen Y, Liu M, Bi C, Jiang C, Iqbal J, McKeithan TW, Chan WC, Ding SJ, Fu K. Quantitative proteomics reveals that miR-155 regulates the PI3K-AKT pathway in diffuse large B-cell lymphoma. Am J Pathol. 2012;181(1):26–33. DOI: 10.1016/j.ajpath. 2012.03.013.

[291] Willimott S, Wagner SD. miR-125b and miR-155 contribute to BCL2 repression and proliferation in response to CD40 ligand (CD154) in human leukemic B-cells. J Biol Chem. 2012 Jan 20;287(4):2608–17. doi: 10.1074/jbc.M111.285718.

[292] Rai D, Kim SW, McKeller MR, Dahia PL, Aguiar RC. Targeting of SMAD5 links microRNA-155 to the TGF-beta pathway and lymphomagenesis. Proc Natl Acad Sci U S A. 2010;107(7):3111–6. DOI: 10.1073/pnas.0910667107.

[293] Kong W, He L, Coppola M, Guo J, Esposito NN, Coppola D, Cheng JQ. MicroRNA-155 regulates cell survival, growth, and chemosensitivity by targeting FOXO3a in breast cancer. J Biol Chem. 2010;285(23):17869–79. DOI: 10.1074/jbc.M110.101055.

[294] Jiang S, Zhang HW, Lu MH, He XH, Li Y, Gu H, Liu MF, Wang ED. MicroRNA-155 functions as an OncomiR in breast cancer by targeting the suppressor of cytokine signaling 1 gene. Cancer Res. 2010;70(8):3119–27. DOI: 10.1158/0008-5472.CAN-09-4250.

[295] Inomata M, Tagawa H, Guo YM, Kameoka Y, Takahashi N, Sawada K. MicroRNA-17-92 down-regulates expression of distinct targets in different B-cell lymphoma subtypes. Blood. 2009;113(2):396–402. DOI: 10.1182/blood-2008-07-163907.

[296] Venturini L, Battmer K, Castoldi M, Schultheis B, Hochhaus A, Muckenthaler MU, Ganser A, Eder M, Scherr M. Expression of the miR-17-92 polycistron in chronic

myeloid leukemia (CML) CD34+ cells. Blood. 2007;109(10):4399–405. DOI: http://dx.doi.org/10.1182/blood-2006-09-045104.

[297] He L, Thomson JM, Hemann MT, Hernando-Monge E, Mu D, Goodson S, Powers S, Cordon-Cardo C, Lowe SW, Hannon GJ, Hammond SM. A microrna polycistron as a potential human oncogene. Nature. 2005;435:828–833. DOI: 10.1038/nature03552.

[298] Mu P, Han YC, Betel D, Yao E, Squatrito M, Ogrodowski P, de Stanchina E, D'Andrea A, Sander C, Ventura A. Genetic dissection of the mir-17B92 cluster of micrornas in myc-induced b-cell lymphomas. Genes Dev. 2009;23:2806–2811. DOI: 10.1101/gad.1872909.

[299] Conkrite K, Sundby M, Mukai S, Thomson JM, Mu D, Hammond SM, MacPherson D. Mir-17B92 cooperates with rb pathway mutations to promote retinoblastoma. Genes Dev. 2011;25:1734–1745. DOI: 10.1101/gad.17027411.

[300] Dews M, Homayouni A, Yu D, Murphy D, Sevignani C, Wentzel E, Furth EE, Lee WM, Enders GH, Mendell JT, Thomas-Tikhonenko A. Augmentation of tumor angiogenesis by a myc-activated microrna cluster. Nat Genet. 2006;38:1060–1065. DOI: 10.1038/ng1855.

[301] Leivonen SK, Mäkelä R, Ostling P, Kohonen P, Haapa-Paananen S, Kleivi K, Enerly E, Aakula A, Hellström K, Sahlberg N, Kristensen VN, Børresen-Dale AL, Saviranta P, Perälä M, Kallioniemi O. Protein lysate microarray analysis to identify micrornas regulating estrogen receptor signaling in breast cancer cell lines. Oncogene. 2009;28:3926–3936. DOI: 10.1038/onc.2009.241.

[302] Taguchi A, Yanagisawa K, Tanaka M, Cao K, Matsuyama Y, Goto H, Takahashi T. Identification of hypoxia-inducible factor-1 alpha as a novel target for miR-17-92 microRNA cluster. Cancer Res. 2008;68(14):5540–5. DOI: 10.1158/0008-5472.CAN-07-6460.

[303] Ebi H, Sato T, Sugito N, Hosono Y, Yatabe Y, Matsuyama Y, Yamaguchi T, Osada H, Suzuki M, Takahashi T. Counterbalance between RB inactivation and miR-17-92 overexpression in reactive oxygen species and DNA damage induction in lung cancers. Oncogene. 2009;28(38):3371–9. DOI: 10.1038/onc.2009.201.

[304] Osada H, Takahashi T. Let-7 and mir-17-92: Small-sized major players in lung cancer development. Cancer Sci. 2011;102:9–17. DOI: 10.1111/j.1349-7006.2010.01707.x.

[305] Smith AL, Iwanaga R, Drasin DJ, Micalizzi DS, Vartuli RL, Tan AC, Ford HL. The miR-106b-25 cluster targets Smad7, activates TGF-β signaling, and induces EMT and tumor initiating cell characteristics downstream of Six1 in human breast cancer. Oncogene. 2012;31(50):5162–71. DOI: 10.1038/onc.2012.11.

[306] Petrocca F, Visone R, Onelli MR, Shah MH, Nicoloso MS, de Martino I, Iliopoulos D, Pilozzi E, Liu CG, Negrini M, Cavazzini L, Volinia S, Alder H, Ruco LP, Baldassarre G, Croce CM, Vecchione A.E2F1-regulated microRNAs impair TGFbeta-dependent

cell-cycle arrest and apoptosis in gastric cancer. Cancer Cell. 2008;13(3):272–86. DOI: 10.1016/j.ccr.2008.02.013.

[307] He Y, Cui Y, Wang W, Gu J, Guo S, Ma K, Luo X. Hypomethylation of the hsa-miR-191 locus causes high expression of hsa-mir-191 and promotes the epithelial-to-mesenchymal transition in hepatocellular carcinoma. Neoplasia. 2011;13(9):841–53. DOI: 10.1593/neo.11698.

[308] Elyakim E, Sitbon E, Faerman A, Tabak S, Montia E, Belanis L, Dov A, Marcusson EG, Bennett CF, Chajut A, Cohen D, Yerushalmi N.hsa-miR-191 is a candidate oncogene target for hepatocellular carcinoma therapy. Cancer Res. 2010;70(20):8077–87. DOI: 10.1158/0008-5472.CAN-10-1313.

[309] Shi X, Su S, Long J, Mei B, Chen Y. MicroRNA-191 targets N-deacetylase/N-sulfotransferase 1 and promotes cell growth in human gastric carcinoma cell line MGC803. Acta Biochim Biophys Sin (Shanghai). 2011;43(11):849-56. DOI: 10.1093/abbs/gmr084.

[310] Dongfang Wang, Jin Gu, Ting Wang, Zijian Ding. OncomiRDB: A database for the experimentally verified oncogenic and tumor-suppressive microRNAs. Bioinformatics. 2014:30(15):2237–2238. DOI: 10.1093/bioinformatics/btu155.

Chapter 2

Cell Cycle Regulation via the p53, PTEN, and BRCA1 Tumor Suppressors

Akari Minami, Toshiyuki Murai, Atsuko Nakanishi,
Yasuko Kitagishi, Mayuko Ichimura and
Satoru Matsuda

Additional information is available at the end of the chapter

http://dx.doi.org/10.5772/61116

Abstract

Multiple cell cycle regulatory proteins play an important role in oncogenesis. Cancer cells may arise from dysregulation of various genes involved in the regulation of the cell cycle. In addition, cyclin-dependent kinase inhibitors are regarded as key regulators for cancer cell proliferation. Accordingly, permission of impaired cells by cell cycle checkpoints suppresses carcinogenesis. P53, a multifunctional protein, controls G1-S transition, which is the strongest tumor suppressor involved in the regulation of cell cycle. The p53 is stimulated by cellular stress like oxidative stress. Upon activation, p53 leads to cell cycle arrest and promotes DNA repair; otherwise, it induces apoptosis. One of the target effectors of p53 is the phosphatase and tensin homolog deleted on chromosome 10 (PTEN). The tumor suppressor PTEN is a dual-specificity phosphatase which has protein phosphatase activity and lipid phosphatase activity that antagonizes PI3K/AKT activity. The PI3K/AKT cell survival pathway is shown as regulator of cell proliferation. The p53 cooperates with PTEN and might be an essential barrier in development of cancers. BRCA1 plays an important role in DNA repair processes related to maintenance of genomic integrity and control of cell growth. The inactivation of these tumor suppressor proteins confers a growth advantage of cancer. This chapter summarizes the function of several tumor suppressors in the cell cycle regulation.

Keywords: p53, PTEN, BRCA1, AKT, MDM2, p21WAF1, protein interaction, protein expression, cell signaling, DNA repair, cell cycle regulation

1. Introduction

Mechanisms of cell cycle are predominantly controlled by p53 tumor suppressor [1, 2]. The p53 transcription factor can bring G1 arrest of the cell cycle by transactivating several downstream molecules [3, 4], which regulates various signaling pathways involved in the cellular response to genome stress and DNA damage. Through the stress-induced activation, p53 triggers the expression of target genes that protect the genetic reliability of cells [5]. Germinal mutations of the *p53* gene constitute an etiological base of Li-Fraumeni syndrome, which is a sporadic heterogeneous autosomal dominant inherited oncogenic disorder [6]. BRCA1, a famous breast cancer tumor suppressor, is associated with breast and ovarian cancer risk and genetic susceptibility [7]. Studies have shown that p53 as well as BRCA1 plays a key role in DNA damage responses [8]. In addition, BRCA1 could work together with phosphatase and tensin homolog deleted in chromosome 10 (*PTEN*), which is also a tumor suppressor gene that is deleted or mutated in a range of human cancers [7, 9], and may be a critical protection in development of several tumors [7, 9]. Actually, PI3K/AKT pathway is constitutively active in BRCA1 defective human cancer cells [10]. Both *PTEN* and *BRCA1* genes are documented as one of the most frequently deleted and/or mutated in various human cancers. Loss or decrease of these PTEN or BRCA1 activities, by either mutation or reduced expression, seems to have a critical role in various cancer developments. PTEN prevents the activation of PI3K/AKT pathway by dephosphorylating the membrane phospholipid PIP3 [11]. Loss of PTEN results in increased AKT recruitment to the plasma membrane and stimulates the signaling pathway. Mutations in *PTEN* genome are the cause of distinctive hamartoma syndromes (*PTEN*-related Proteus syndrome, Cowden syndrome, Proteus-like syndrome, Bannayan-Riley-Ruvalcaba syndrome) with higher risk for a development of several tumors [12]. Furthermore, *BRCA1* and *PTEN* have been shown to be involved in a complex linkage on the interaction with the p53 as presented in Figure 1. Although they are functionally distinct, mutual cooperation has been proposed. These tumor suppressors regulate diverse cellular activities including DNA damage repair, cell cycle arrest, cell differentiation, cell proliferation, cell migration, and cell apoptosis [13]. Importantly, mutations in all of these genes have been associated with increased risk of developing cancers. This review summarizes the function of the tumor suppressors in DNA repair and cell cycle regulation. We will also discuss the role of cellular signaling through protein interaction pathways for the potential implications in the fundamental DNA repair and cell cycle regulation.

2. Characteristics of *p53*, *PTEN*, and *BRCA1*

The *p53* gene encodes a nuclear 393-amino-acid protein which is a transcription factor (Figure 2). The p53 tumor suppressor plays an essential role in regulating cellular processes including cell cycle arrest, apoptosis, cell metabolism, and cell senescence. Inactivation of *p53* gene is related to the development of most types of cancers [14], suggesting that *p53* also plays a critical role in preventing normal cells to becoming cancer cells. In addition, importance of *p53* as an inherited cancer susceptibility gene has been revealed in the Li-Fraumeni syndrome [15].

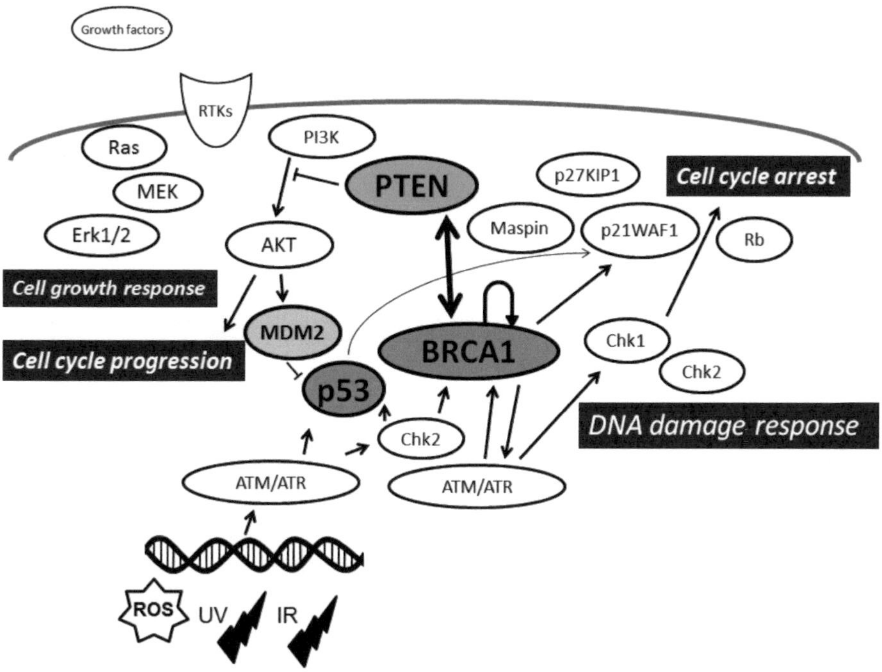

Figure 1. Schematic illustration of the integrative signaling model of tumor suppressors including p53, PTEN, and BRCA1 is shown. Typical examples of molecules known to act on the cell proliferation, DNA damage response, and cell cycle regulation via the regulatory pathway are shown. Note that some critical pathways have been omitted for clarity.

Multiple mechanisms have been shown to accomplish the regulation of p53 activity, which controls the selectivity of p53 for specific transcriptional targets [16]. Discharge of p53 from normal repression by binding with molecules such as MdmX or Mdm2 may be a crucial step in the activation of p53 [17, 18]. Functional activation of p53 links with its higher DNA-binding ability, transcriptional activation, then increased expression of the target genes of p53, which are all related to cell cycle regulation and/or cellular apoptosis.

PTEN tumor suppressor gene is also frequently deleted and mutated in several human cancers [19]. The gene product is a 53-kDa protein with homology to tensin and protein tyrosine phosphatases. Human genomic locus of the *PTEN* consists of 9 exons on chromosome 10q23.3 encoding a 5.5-kb mRNA that postulates a 403-amino-acid open reading frame [20]. Schematic construction of the predicted PTEN protein is presented in Figure 2. The PTEN protein consists of amino-terminal phosphatase, carboxyl-terminal C2, and PDZ (PSD-95, DLG1, and ZO-1) binding domains [21]. The structure offers PTEN with its preference for acidic phospholipid substrates including phosphatidylinositol 3,4,5-triphosphate (PIP3), as the PTEN CX5R(S/T) motif resides within an active site that surrounds the catalytic core with three basic residues, which are critical for PTEN lipid phosphatase activity [22]. PTEN negatively regulates the activity of PI3K/AKT signaling through converting PIP3 into phosphatidylinositol 4,5-bisphosphate (PIP2) [23]. PIP3 is the principal second messenger of the PI3K pathway that

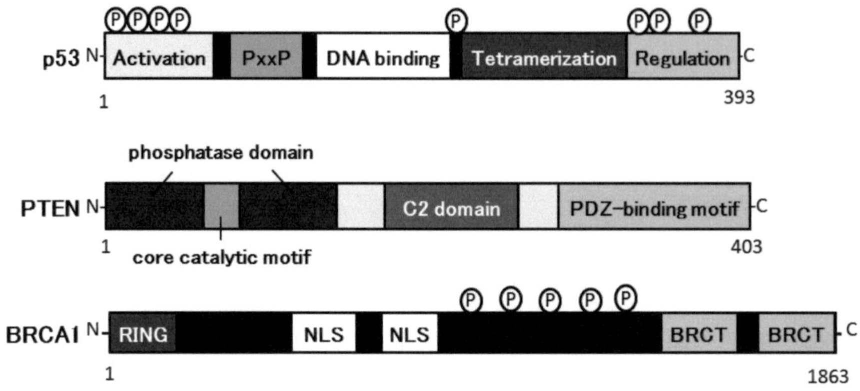

Figure 2. Schematic structures of p53, PTEN, and BRCA1 proteins are shown. The predicted consensual domain structures for each protein are depicted. The functionally key sites including the sites of protein phosphorylation are shown. Note that the sizes of protein are modified for clarity. Activation = transactivation domain; PxxP = proline-rich region; RING = (Really Interesting New Gene) finger domain, NLS = Nuclear Localization Signal, BRCT = BRCA1 C Terminus; C2 domain = a protein structural domain involved in targeting proteins to cell membranes; PDZ = a common structural domain in signaling proteins (PSD95, Dlg, ZO-1, etc.)

mediates receptor tyrosine kinase (RTK) signaling to the cell survival kinase AKT. In general, growth factors stimulate RTKs, then activate PI3K and AKT. Upon activation, the inositol ring phosphorylated by PI3K serves to fix AKT to the plasma membrane, where it is sequentially phosphorylated and completely activated by 3-phosphoinositide-dependent kinases PDK1 and PDK2 [24]. Subsequently, activated AKT phosphorylates target proteins involved in cell survival, cell cycling, proliferation, and cell migration [25]. PTEN may act as a regulator of keeping basal levels of PIP3 under a threshold for those signaling activation. Overexpression of PTEN inhibits cell growth by supporting cell cycle arrest, which requires the lipid phosphatase activity of PTEN [26], which correlates with reduced levels and nuclear localization of cyclin-D1 [27], an important molecule of cell cycle regulated by PTEN and AKT. In addition, PTEN induces the cell cycle arrest by upregulating the cell cycle inhibitor p27KIP1 [28]. However, studies have shown many tumor suppressive activities for PTEN that are working within the nucleus, where catalysis of PIP3 does not appear to characterize a main function of the enzyme. The nuclear PTEN activities may include the regulation of genomic stability and several gene expression, indeed despite that the central role of PTEN is as a negative regulator of the PI3K pathway. PTEN activity can be regulated by posttranslational regulation including phosphorylation, oxidation, and acetylation [29, 30].

BRCA1 cDNA encodes for 1863-amino-acid protein with two nuclear localization signals (NLS) and an amino terminal conserved RING finger motif which is the shared motif present in E3 ubiquitin ligases [31] (Figure 2). The RING finger domain interacts with E2 ubiquitin ligases and applies E3 ligase activity [32]. Knock-in mice with deficient BRCA1 activity exhibit diverse genomic instability and tumor-forming phenotypes [33]. Exon 11 encodes an unstructured region of the BRCA1 protein that is phosphorylated by the ATM and Chk2 kinases in a DNA-damage-dependent manner [34, 35], and the specific function of BRCA1 may be regulated by phosphorylation. BRCA1 becomes more phosphorylated after exposure to the DNA-damaging agents [36]. The carboxyl-terminal domain of BRCA1 is involved in association with specific phosphorylated proteins [37]. Because BRCA1 plays a crucial role in maintaining genome stability, the mutation of BRCA1 is associated with increased genomic instability in cells, which consequently accelerates the mutation rate of the other critical genes. Inherited BRCA1 germline mutation is revealed as a genetic susceptibility leading to high risk of breast and ovarian cancers [38]. Although *BRCA1* gene mutations are rare in breast and/or ovarian cancers, BRCA1 protein expression is often decreased in sporadic cancer specimens. Principally, the role of BRCA1 in cell cycle control has been understood by its ability to interact with various cyclin proteins and various cyclin-dependent kinases [39, 40].

3. Relationship among PTEN, p53, BRCA1, and MDM2

The PTEN and p53 complex augments the p53-DNA binding and the transcriptional action [41], which may upregulate the expression of PTEN itself and p21WAF1, which is a key molecule involved in cell cycle arrest [42]. Indeed, a superior function of p53 is to work as a transcription factor by attaching to the definite DNA consensus sequence on the p53 responsive genes. Consequently, p53 indirectly inhibits production of PIP3 by inducing the expression of this PTEN. In addition, PTEN associates with p53 and regulates the transcriptional activity of p53 by modulating its DNA binding. PTEN is also required for the maintenance of p53 acetylation [43], which is essential for target gene transcription. An adjacent function of PTEN as a tumor suppressor is accomplished through the stabilization of the p53 protein. PTEN and p53 form a complex in the nucleus under hypoxic conditions [44]. Nuclear PTEN is sufficient to reduce cancer progression in a p53-dependent manner [45]. In addition, the nuclear PTEN seems to mediate DNA damage repair through modulating the activity of DNA repair molecules. The PI3K-dependent activation of AKT indirectly leads to the inhibition of p53 functions by activating another tumor suppressor MDM2 [46]. Activation of AKT has the potential of reducing the p53-mediated cell cycle checkpoints through phosphorylation and appropriation of p21WAF1 [47]. By the way, several PI3K inhibitors favorably reduce proliferation of BRCA1-defective breast cancer cells. For example, BEZ235 inhibits not only PI3K/mTOR but also ATM/ATR [48, 49]. It is possible that ATM pathways are involved in upregulation of the PI3K/AKT pathway in BRCA1-defective cancer cells. In contrast, BRCA1 may regulate the PI3K/AKT pathway by acting on upstream kinases of AKT. Overexpression of wild-type BRCA1 could further reduce basal phosphorylation of AKT levels in MCF7 cells [10, 50]. In addition, reduced levels of PTEN are associated with radio-resistance which can be suppressed by the ectopic PTEN expression [51, 52].

MDM2 controls carcinogenesis, whose mRNA level is also transcriptionally regulated by p53 in response to DNA damage [53]. MDM2 protein and subcellular localization are post-translationally modulated by AKT [53]. Besides inhibiting the PI3K/AKT signaling, PTEN also promotes translocation of the MDM2 into the nucleus. Furthermore, PTEN modulates *MDM2* transcription by negatively regulating its promoter [41]. PTEN controls *MDM2* promoter activity through its lipid phosphatase activity, independent of the p53 activity [53]. In *PTEN*-

null cells, *MDM2* promoter activity is upregulated, resulting in increased *MDM2* expression [53]. MDM2 also regulates the activity of p53 protein by transferring the nuclear p53 protein into the cytoplasm and by promoting the degradation of the p53 protein [54]. PTEN upregulates the p53 level as well as its activity by downregulating *MDM2* transcription [55]. However, in the absence of p53, PTEN may have a role in inhibiting MDM2-mediated carcinogenesis through regulation of *MDM2* transcription. The p53 and MDM2 complex transports from the nucleus into the cytoplasm, where MDM2 serves as an E3 ubiquitin ligase [56]. Therefore, p53 and MDM2 form a regulatory feedback loop in which p53 positively regulates MDM2 activity. Inactivation of either gene should result in lower protein levels of the other gene. The ability of PTEN to inhibit the nuclear entry of MDM2 increases the cellular content. The BRCA1 carboxyl-terminal region can also stimulate transcription of the p53-responsive promoter of MDM2 [57]. BRCA1 has been shown to affect the gene transcription, but how it does so remains elusive. Essentially, the most important molecule for the DNA damage recognition may be ATM, which is a key checkpoint kinase that phosphorylates various proteins including BRCA1 and/or p53 in response to the DNA damage [58]. BRCA1 activates the CDK inhibitor p21WAF1 and the p53 tumor suppressor protein, which regulates several genes that control the cell cycle checkpoints [59, 60]. Inhibition of this important DNA repair pathway seems to block the mechanisms that are required for normal cell survival in the presence of oncogenic mutations due to DNA damage.

4. Involvement of the p53-PTEN-MDM2-BRCA1 loop in cell cycle regulation

The levels of p53 could vary and is positively related to the amount of DNA damage [61]. Low levels of p53 may induce cell cycle arrest, whereas high levels of p53 may induce apoptosis. On the other hand, growth factor-activated AKT signaling supports progression of cell cycle by acting on several factors involved in the G1/S or G2/M cell cycle transitions. Because the ability of p53 to induce cell cycle arrest and/or cell apoptosis can be provoked by cell survival signals including the AKT pathway, the cell growth signal circuitously leads to the inhibition of p53 by triggering its negative regulators [62]. The p53 protein also regulates BRCA1 transcription both in vitro and in vivo, and BRCA1 participates in p53 accumulation after irradiation through regulation of its phosphorylation and MDM2 expression [63]. MDM2 can act as a modifier of BRCA1 mutant and may accelerate breast and ovarian carcinogenesis [64]. In addition, p53 and PTEN are known to interact and to regulate each other at the transcription as well as protein level, which could be at the important control machinery for switching between survival and death. Given the ability of PTEN to stabilize p53 protein through provoking the AKT-MDM2 complex or by increasing p53 acetylation, the decreased p53 activity in PTEN-lacking tumor cells could be plausible. PTEN and BRCA1 may be regulated and interact with each other at multiple levels including transcription, protein modulation, and protein stability. Therefore, the p53-PTEN-MDM2-BRCA1 loop in cell cycle regulation now becomes dominant (Figure 3). These cross talks are frequently a combination of reciprocally antagonistic pathways, which may often serve as an additional regulatory effect on the

http://dx.doi.org/10.5772/61116

expression of key genes involved in cell cycle and carcinogenesis. Interestingly, genistein, which is a soy isoflavone, brings regulation between PTEN and p53 to support cell cycle arrest [65]. Genistein induces PTEN expression and nuclear accumulation, which elicits a sequence of PTEN-dependent nuclear p53 accumulation and recruitment of the PTEN/p53 complex to the p53 binding sites [65], then attenuates expression of cell proliferative genes [65]. In addition, genistein inhibits cell proliferation and induces cell apoptosis more proficiently in BRCA1-mutant cells than in cells expressing wild-type BRCA1 protein [66]. BRCA1-mutant breast cancer cells are highly sensitive to genistein treatment, and AKT could be genistein targets in these cells [66]. Accordingly, genetic variants in the molecules of p53, PTEN, BRCA1, and MDM2 may play roles in tumor suppressor network mediating a susceptibility to cancer. Remarkably, it has also been presented that zinc deficiency modulates the p53-PTEN-BRCA1-MDM2 signaling network in normal cells [67].

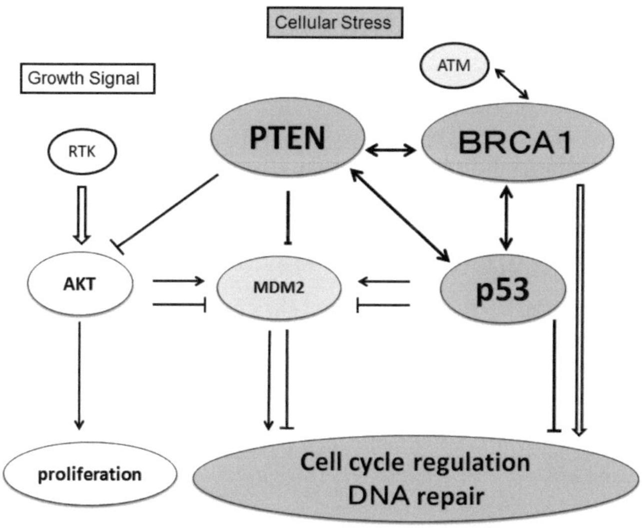

Figure 3. Suggestion of various regulatory loops involving the p53-PTEN-MDM2-BRCA1 network on cell cycle regulation. Interactions are shown as arrows to mean activation, while hammerheads, to mean inhibition. Expression of these tumor suppressor genes is regulated by genetic, epigenetic, and transcriptional changes, which may result in the DNA repair and cell cycle regulation in a cell. Downregulation of the function can contribute to genomic instability, which promotes malignant transformation of cells. Note that some critical pathways have been omitted for clarity.

5. Perspective

In unstressed cells, p53 may be regularly kept at low levels by its negative regulator MDM2. This feedback loop among the p53-PTEN-MDM2-BRCA1 may function for the accurate regulation of the DNA repair and cell cycle (Figure 3). When stressed, the tumor suppressor p53 predominantly induces cell cycle arrest or apoptosis in the response to DNA damage. Indeed, the regulation is crucial for the effective design of novel cancer therapeutics. Further mechanistic studies are needed in order to understand the exact molecular mechanisms for the effective treatment of cancers with the functional alterations in the cellular signaling loop. Targets within this pathway could provide strategies therapeutically valuable for several cancer treatments. It is important to investigate the linkage among the molecules, and elucidation of interaction-specific functions may provide insight into regulatory aspects of these tumor suppressors as well as opportunities for therapeutic intervention. Such molecular interactions may sustain the biological plausibility that the combination of variants of the p53-PTEN-MDM2-BRCA1 network could result in more comprehensive. Genetic analysis for germline mutations in these key genes allows for the identification of characters at increased risk of cancers. However, they may be regulated and interact with each other at multiple levels including transcription, protein modulation, and protein stability. Obviously, understanding the regulation is crucial for the effective design of novel cancer prevention and therapeutics. Further studies are needed to understand molecular mechanisms in more detail.

6. Abbreviations

ATM: ataxia telangiectasia-mutated

BRCA1: breast cancer susceptibility gene 1

HDM2: human homolog of MDM2

LOH: Loss of heterozygosity

MDM2: murine double minute 2

NEDL1: NEDD4-like ubiquitin protein ligase-1

NF-κB: nuclear factor kappaB

NLS: Nuclear Localization Signal

mTOR: mammalian target of rapamycin

PDZ: PSD-95, DLG1, and ZO-1

PEST: proline, glutamic acid, serine and threonine

PTEN: phosphatase and tensin homolog deleted on chromosome 10

PIP2: phosphatidylinositol 4,5- bisphosphate

PIP3: phosphatidylinositol 3,4,5-triphosphate

PI3K: phosphoinositide-3 kinase

RING: really interesting new gene finger domain

RTK: receptor tyrosine kinase

ROS: reactive oxidative species

http://dx.doi.org/10.5772/61116

Acknowledgements

This work was supported by JSPS KAKENHI Grant Number 25560050, 26-12035, 24240098.

Author details

Akari Minami[1], Toshiyuki Murai[2], Atsuko Nakanishi[1], Yasuko Kitagishi[1], Mayuko Ichimura[1] and Satoru Matsuda[1*]

*Address all correspondence to: smatsuda@cc.nara-wu.ac.jp

1 Department of Food Science and Nutrition, Nara Women's University, Kita-Uoya Nishimachi, Nara, Japan

2 Department of Microbiology and Immunology and Department of Genome Biology, Graduate School of Medicine, Osaka University, -2 Yamada-oka, Suita, Japan

Akari Minami and Satoru Matsuda contributed equally to this work.
Competing interests statement: The authors declare that they have no competing financial interests.

References

[1] Xia L, Paik A, Li JJ (2004). p53 activation in chronic radiation-treated breast cancer cells: regulation of MDM2/p14ARF. Cancer Res. 64:221–228.

[2] Calcagno DQ, Freitas VM, Leal MF, de Souza CR, Demachki S, Montenegro R, Assumpção PP, Khayat AS, Smith Mde A, dos Santos AK, Burbano RR (2013). MYC, FBXW7 and TP53 copy number variation and expression in gastric cancer. BMC Gastroenterol. 13:141.

[3] Kuribayashi K, El-Deiry WS (2008). Regulation of programmed cell death by the p53 pathway. Adv Exp Med Biol. 615:201–221.

[4] Matsumoto M, Furihata M, Ohtsuki Y (2006). Posttranslational phosphorylation of mutant p53protein in tumor development. Med Mol Morphol. 39(2):79–87.

[5] Frum RA, Grossman SR (2014). Mechanisms of mutant p53 stabilization in cancer. Subcell Biochem. 85:187–197.

[6] Merino D, Malkin D (2014). p53 and hereditary cancer. Subcell Biochem. 85:1–16.

[7] Minami A, Nakanishi A, Ogura Y, Kitagishi Y, Matsuda S (2014). Connection between tumor suppressor BRCA1 and PTEN in damaged DNA repair. Front Oncol. 4:318.

[8] Yang X, Zhang Z, Wang X, Wang Y, Zhang X, Lu H, Wang SL (2013). Cytochrome P450 2A13 enhances the sensitivity of human bronchial epithelial cells to aflatoxin B1-induced DNA damage. Toxicol Appl Pharmacol. 270:114–121.

[9] Zhou C, Smith JL, Liu J (2003). Role of BRCA1 in cellular resistance to paclitaxel and ionizing radiation in an ovarian cancer cell line carrying a defective BRCA1. Oncogene. 22:2396–2404.

[10] Yi YW, Kang HJ, Kim HJ, Hwang JS, Wang A, Bae I (2013). Inhibition of constitutively activated phosphoinositide 3-kinase/AKT pathway enhances antitumor activity of chemotherapeutic agents in breast cancer susceptibility gene 1-defective breast cancer cells. Mol Carcinog. 52:667–675.

[11] Carnero A, Paramio JM (2014). The PTEN/PI3K/AKT pathway in vivo, cancer mouse models. Front Oncol. 4:252.

[12] Spinelli L, Black FM, Berg JN, Eickholt BJ, Leslie NR (2015). Functionally distinct groups of inherited PTEN mutations in autism and tumour syndromes. J Med Genet. 52:128–134.

[13] Yu X, Si J, Zhang Y, Dewille JW (2010). CCAAT/enhancer binding protein-delta (C/EBP-delta) regulates cell growth, migration and differentiation. Cancer Cell Int. 10:48.

[14] Kim E, Giese A, Deppert W (2009). Wild-type p53 in cancer cells: when a guardian turns into a blackguard. Biochem Pharmacol. 77:11–20.

[15] Tomkova K, Tomka M, Zajac V (2008). Contribution of p53, p63, and p73 to the developmental diseases and cancer. Neoplasma. 55:177–181.

[16] Cheok CF, Lane DP (2012). Seeking synergy in p53transcriptional activation for cancer therapy. Discov Med. 14:263–271.

[17] Wade M, Li YC, Wahl GM (2013). MDM2, MDMX and p53 in oncogenesis and cancer therapy. Nat Rev Cancer. 13:83–96.

[18] Zhang Q, Zeng SX, Lu H (2014). Targeting p53-MDM2-MDMX loop for cancer therapy. Subcell Biochem. 85:281–319.

[19] Carracedo A, Alimonti A, Pandolfi PP (2011). PTEN level in tumor suppression: how much is too little? Cancer Res. 71:629–633.

[20] Eng C (2003). PTEN: one gene, many syndromes. Hum Mutat. 22:183–198.

[21] Sotelo NS, Schepens JT, Valiente M, Hendriks WJ, Pulido R (2015). PTEN-PDZ domain interactions: binding of PTEN to PDZ domains of PTPN13. Methods. 77–78:147–156.

[22] Maehama T, Taylor GS, Dixon JE (2001). PTEN and myotubularin: novel phosphoinositide phosphatases. Annu Rev Biochem. 70:247–279.

[23] Miao B, Skidan I, Yang J, Lugovskoy A, Reibarkh M, Long K, Brazell T, Durugkar KA, Maki J, Ramana CV, Schaffhausen B, Wagner G, Torchilin V, Yuan J, Degterev A (2010). Small molecule inhibition of phosphatidylinositol-3,4,5-triphosphate (PIP3) binding to pleckstrin homology domains. Proc Natl Acad Sci U S A. 107:20126–20131.

[24] Fresno Vara JA, Casado E, de Castro J, Cejas P, Belda-Iniesta C, González-Barón M (2004). PI3K/Akt signalling pathway and cancer. Cancer Treat Rev. 30:193–204.

[25] Anai M, Shojima N, Katagiri H, Ogihara T, Sakoda H, Onishi Y, Ono H, Fujishiro M, Fukushima Y, Horike N, Viana A, Kikuchi M, Noguchi N, Takahashi S, Takata K, Oka Y, Uchijima Y, Kurihara H, Asano T (2005). A novel protein kinase B (PKB)/AKT-binding protein enhances PKB kinase activity and regulates DNA synthesis. J Biol Chem. 280:18525–18535.

[26] Petrella BL, Brinckerhoff CE (2009). PTEN suppression of YY1 induces HIF-2 activity in von-Hippel-Lindau-null renal-cell carcinoma. Cancer Biol Ther. 8:1389–1401.

[27] Yamamoto M, Tamakawa S, Yoshie M, Yaginuma Y, Ogawa K (2006). Neoplastic hepatocyte growth associated with cyclin D1 redistribution from the cytoplasm to the nucleus in mouse hepatocarcinogenesis. Mol Carcinog. 45:901–913.

[28] Hennenlotter J, Ohneseit PA, Simon P, Merseburger AS, Serth J, Kuehs U, Kramer M, Hartmann JT, Stenzl A, Kuczyk MA (2008). PTEN and p27Kip1 are not downregulated in the majority of renal cell carcinomas – implications for Akt activation. Oncol Rep. 19:1141–1147.

[29] Tamguney T, Stokoe D (2007). New insights into PTEN. J Cell Sci. 120:4071–4079.

[30] Shi Y, Paluch BE, Wang X, Jiang X (2012). PTEN at a glance. J Cell Sci. 125:4687–4692.

[31] Yang Y, Swaminathan S, Martin BK, Sharan SK (2003). Aberrant splicing induced by missense mutations in BRCA1: clues from a humanized mouse model. Hum Mol Genet. 12:2121–2131.

[32] Miyamoto K (2014). Structural model of ubiquitin transfer onto an artificial RING finger as an E3 ligase. Sci Rep. 4:6574.

[33] Bahassi el M, Penner CG, Robbins SB, Tichy E, Feliciano E, Yin M, Liang L, Deng L, Tischfield JA, Stambrook PJ (2007). The breast cancer susceptibility allele CHEK2*1100delC promotes genomic instability in a knock-in mouse model. Mutat Res. 616:201–209.

[34] Brew CT, Aronchik I, Hsu JC, Sheen JH, Dickson RB, Bjeldanes LF, Firestone GL (2006). Indole-3-carbinol activates the ATM signaling pathway independent of DNA

damage to stabilize p53 and induce G1 arrest of human mammary epithelial cells. Int J Cancer. 118:857–868.

[35] Li J, Stern DF (2005). DNA damage regulates Chk2 association with chromatin. J Biol Chem. 280:37948–37956.

[36] Lane TF (2004). BRCA1 and transcription. Cancer Biol Ther. 3:528–533.

[37] Yu X, Chini CC, He M, Mer G, Chen J (2003). The BRCT domain is a phospho-protein binding domain. Science. 302:639–642.

[38] Fourati A, Louchez MM, Fournier J, Gamoudi A, Rahal K, El May MV, El May A, Revillion F, Peyrat JP (2014). Screening for common mutations in BRCA1 and BRCA2 genes: interest in genetic testing of Tunisian families with breast and/or ovarian cancer. Bull Cancer. 101:E36–E40.

[39] Jhanwar-Uniyal M (2003). BRCA1 in cancer, cell cycle and genomic stability. Front Biosci. 8:s1107–s1117.

[40] Krämer A, Lukas J, Bartek J (2004). Checking out the centrosome. Cell Cycle. 3:1390–1393.

[41] Freeman DJ, Li AG, Wei G, Li HH, Kertesz N, Lesche R, Whale AD, Martinez-Diaz H, Rozengurt N, Cardiff RD, Liu X, Wu H (2003). PTEN tumor suppressor regulates p53 protein levels and activity through phosphatase-dependent and -independent mechanisms. Cancer Cell. 3:117–130.

[42] Todorova VK, Kaufmann Y, Luo S, Klimberg VS (2006). Modulation of p53 and c-myc in DMBA-induced mammary tumors by oral glutamine. Nutr Cancer. 54:263–273.

[43] Li AG, Piluso LG, Cai X, Wei G, Sellers WR, Liu X (2006). Mechanistic insights into maintenance of high p53acetylation by PTEN. Mol Cell. 23:575–587.

[44] Eitel JA, Bijangi-Vishehsaraei K, Saadatzadeh MR, Bhavsar JR, Murphy MP, Pollok KE, Mayo LD (2009). PTEN and p53 are required for hypoxia induced expression of maspin in glioblastoma cells. Cell Cycle. 8:896–901.

[45] Chang CJ, Mulholland DJ, Valamehr B, Mosessian S, Sellers WR, Wu H (2008). PTEN nuclear localization is regulated by oxidative stress and mediates p53-dependent tumor suppression. Mol Cell Biol. 28:3281–3289.

[46] Fenouille N, Puissant A, Tichet M, Zimniak G, Abbe P, Mallavialle A, Rocchi S, Ortonne JP, Deckert M, Ballotti R, Tartare-Deckert S (2011). SPARC functions as an anti-stress factor by inactivating p53 through Akt-mediated MDM2 phosphorylation to promote melanoma cell survival. Oncogene. 30:4887–4900.

[47] Mitsuuchi Y, Johnson SW, Selvakumaran M, Williams SJ, Hamilton TC, Testa JR (2000). The phosphatidylinositol 3-kinase/AKT signal transduction pathway plays a

critical role in the expression of p21WAF1/CIP1/SDI1 induced by cisplatin and paclitaxel. Cancer Res. 60:5390–5394.

[48] Sun Z, Li Q, Zhang S, Chen J, Huang L, Ren J, Chang Y, Liang Y, Wu G (2015). NVP-BEZ235 overcomes gefitinib-acquired resistance by down-regulating PI3K/AKT/mTOR phosphorylation. Onco Targets Ther. 8:269–277.

[49] Fiskus W, Verstovsek S, Manshouri T, Smith JE, Peth K, Abhyankar S, McGuirk J, Bhalla KN (2013). Dual PI3K/AKT/mTOR inhibitor BEZ235 synergistically enhances the activity of JAK2 inhibitor against cultured and primary human myeloproliferative neoplasm cells. Mol Cancer Ther. 12:577–588.

[50] Nair HB, Perla RP, Kirma NB, Krishnegowda NK, Ganapathy M, Rajhans R, Nair SS, Saikumar P, Vadlamudi RK, Tekmal RR (2012). Estrogen receptor-beta mediates the protective effects of aromatase induction in the MMTV-Her-2/neu x aromatase double transgenic mice. Horm Cancer. 3:26–36.

[51] Ettl T, Viale-Bouroncle S, Hautmann MG, Gosau M, Kölbl O, Reichert TE, Morsczeck C (2015). AKT and MET signalling mediates antiapoptotic radioresistance in head neck cancer cell lines. Oral Oncol. 51:158–163.

[52] Tomioka A, Tanaka M, De Velasco MA, Anai S, Takada S, Kushibiki T, Tabata Y, Rosser CJ, Uemura H, Hirao Y (2008). Delivery of PTEN via a novel gene microcapsule sensitizes prostate cancer cells to irradiation. Mol Cancer Ther. 7:1864–1870.

[53] Chang CJ, Freeman DJ, Wu H (2004). PTEN regulates Mdm2 expression through the P1 promoter. J Biol Chem. 279:29841–29848.

[54] Reed SM, Hagen J, Tompkins VS, Thies K, Quelle FW, Quelle DE (2014). Nuclear interactor of ARF and Mdm2 regulates multiple pathways to activate p53. Cell Cycle. 13:1288–1298.

[55] Mitra AK, Jia G, Gangahar DM, Agrawal DK (2009). Temporal PTEN inactivation causes proliferation of saphenous vein smooth muscle cells of human CABG conduits. J Cell Mol Med. 13:177–187.

[56] Jin L, Li C, Xu Y, Wang L, Liu J, Wang D, Hong C, Jiang Z, Ma Y, Chen Q, Yu F (2013). Epigallocatechin gallate promotes p53 accumulation and activity via the inhibition of MDM2-mediated p53 ubiquitination in human lung cancer cells. Oncol Rep. 29:1983–1990.

[57] Nadeau G, Boufaied N, Moisan A, Lemieux KM, Cayanan C, Monteiro AN, Gaudreau L (2000). BRCA1 can stimulate gene transcription by a unique mechanism. EMBO Rep. 1:260–265.

[58] Caldon CE (2014). Estrogen signaling and the DNA damage response in hormone dependent breast cancers. Front Oncol. 4:106.

[59] Zhan Q (2005). Gadd45a, a p53- and BRCA1-regulated stress protein, in cellular response to DNA damage. Mutat Res. 569:133–143.

[60] Chai YL, Cui J, Shao N, Shyam E, Reddy P, Rao VN (1999). The second BRCT domain of BRCA1 proteins interacts with p53 and stimulates transcription from the p21WAF1/CIP1 promoter. Oncogene. 18:263–268.

[61] Hrubá E, Trilecová L, Marvanová S, Krcmár P, Vykopalová L, Milcová A, Líbalová H, Topinka J, Starsíchová A, Soucek K, Vondrácek J, Machala M (2010). Genotoxic polycyclic aromatic hydrocarbons fail to induce the p53-dependent DNA damage response, apoptosis or cell-cycle arrest in human prostate carcinoma LNCaP cells. Toxicol Lett. 197:227–235.

[62] Collado M, Medema RH, Garcia-Cao I, Dubuisson ML, Barradas M, Glassford J, Rivas C, Burgering BM, Serrano M, Lam EW (2000). Inhibition of the phosphoinositide 3-kinase pathway induces a senescence-like arrest mediated by p27Kip1. J Biol Chem. 275:21960–21968.

[63] Xu X, Qiao W, Linke SP, Cao L, Li WM, Furth PA, Harris CC, Deng CX (2001). Genetic interactions between tumor suppressors Brca1 and p53 in apoptosis, cell cycle and tumorigenesis. Nat Genet. 28:266–271.

[64] Yarden RI, Friedman E, Metsuyanim S, Olender T, Ben-Asher E, Papa MZ (2008). MDM2 SNP309 accelerates breast and ovarian carcinogenesis in BRCA1 and BRCA2 carriers of Jewish-Ashkenazi descent. Breast Cancer Res Treat. 111:497–504.

[65] Park CE, Yun H, Lee EB, Min BI, Bae H, Choe W, Kang I, Kim SS, Ha J (2010). The antioxidant effects of genistein are associated with AMP-activated protein kinase activation and PTEN induction in prostate cancer cells. J Med Food. 13:815–820.

[66] Privat M, Aubel C, Arnould S, Communal Y, Ferrara M, Bignon YJ (2010). AKT and p21 WAF1/CIP1 as potential genistein targets in BRCA1-mutant human breast cancer cell lines. Anticancer Res. 30:2049–2054.

[67] Li J, Tan J, Zhuang L, Banerjee B, Yang X, Chau JF, Lee PL, Hande MP, Li B, Yu Q (2007). Ribosomal protein S27-like, a p53-inducible modulator of cell fate in response to genotoxic stress. Cancer Res. 67:11317–11326.

Chapter 3

Epigenetic Mechanisms in Head and Neck Cancer

Julio Cesar Osorio and Andres Castillo

Additional information is available at the end of the chapter

http://dx.doi.org/10.5772/61135

Abstract

Head and neck cancer (HNC) is one of the most prevalent human malignancies, affecting different anatomic sites of the upper aerodigestive tract (UADT) such as the oral cavity, larynx, and naso-, oro-, and hypopharynx. HNC develops through the accumulation of multiple genetic and epigenetic alterations in a multistep process. In this issue, the aim is to describe epigenetic mechanisms behind HNC. The main mechanisms evaluated are DNA methylation, posttranslational histone modification, and noncoding RNAs.

Keywords: Methylation, Histone modification, microRNA, Long non-coding RNAs

1. Introduction

Genetic information flow (transcription, translation, and subsequent protein modification) in a normal cell represents the machine of cell gene expression.[1] Each cell has the same information, but its expression change between different types of cells. The control of gene expression is therefore at the heart of differentiation and development.[1]

In addition to inheriting genetic information, cells inherit chemical modifications that are not encoded in the nucleotide sequence of DNA, and this modification impacts the program of gene expression. This type of modification has been termed epigenetic information.[1]

Epigenetic refers specifically to the study of mitotically and meiotically heritable changes in the control of gene expression that occur without changes in the nucleotide sequence of genome and chromatin.[2]

In both genetic and epigenetic heritage, mitosis distributes genetic information or the chemical modification through the ontogeny. Meiosis distributes genetic information or chemical modification through the formation of gametes. This means that sperm and egg carry genetic and epigenetic information. When the embryo is formed, this information is distributed through the all the cells by mitosis (Figure 1). When it comes to population level, natural selection determines which genetically and epigenetically inherited information is present.

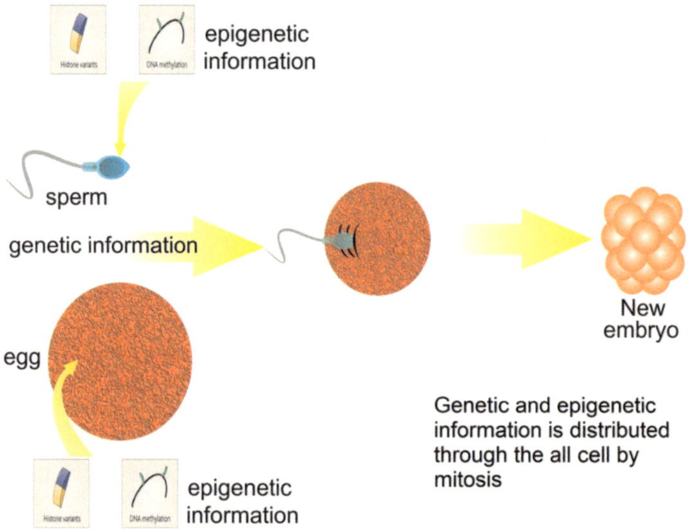

Figure 1. Genetic and epigenetic information in gametes and a new embryo.

Gene regulation and genome function are intimately related to the physical organization of genomic DNA and, in particular, to the way it is packaged into chromatin.[3] There are many chemical modifications affecting DNA, RNA, and proteins that create different epigenetic process.[4] These modifications are related to DNA methylation, histone modifications, chromatin remodeling factors (associated with nucleosome positioning), and noncoding RNAs.[4] The changes will influence the chromatin states and impact gene expression patterns (Figure 2).[5] Epigenetic alterations are associated with chromosomal instability and changes in transcriptional control, which influence the overall gene expression differences seen in many human malignancies.[5]

The carcinogenesis of head and neck cancer (HNC) is a human malignancy influenced by genetic factors, age, geography, and lifestyles, among which include smoking, oral hygiene, and human papillomavirus.[6, 7] In general, different types of carcinogens attack the oral mucosa through the accumulation of multiple genetic and epigenetic alterations in a multistep process.[8] The clinical appearance of HNC preoncogenic lesion of the mucosal surfaces include leukoplakia, erythroplakia, or speckled leukoplakia reflecting the presence of white, red, or mixed white/red lesion, respectively.[9]

HNC is one of the most prevalent human malignancies, affecting different anatomic sites of the upper aerodigestive tract (UADT) such as the oral cavity, larynx, and naso-, oro-, and hypopharynx.[10] The most common histologic type among the head and neck tumors are the squamous cell carcinomas (head and neck squamous cell carcinomas [HNSCCs]).[7]

http://dx.doi.org/10.5772/61135

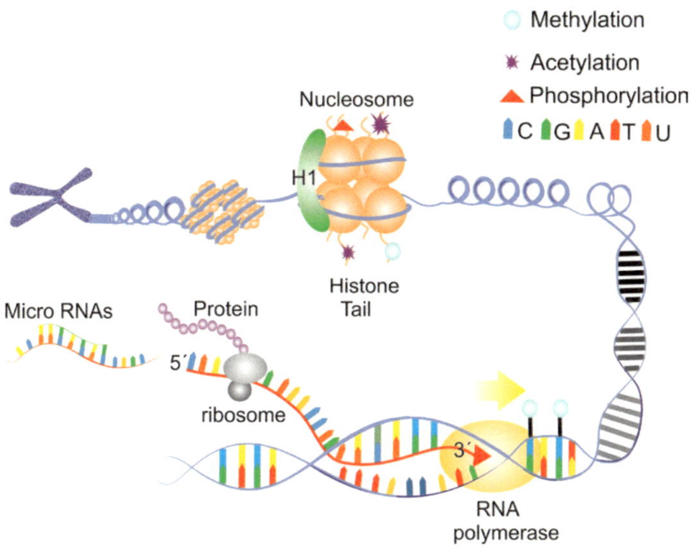

Figure 2. Genetic and epigenetic information.

It was reported that 42,440 new cases of HNSCCs were diagnosed in the United States in 2014, and 8,390 deaths were due to this disease.[11] The mortality rate (from 2003 to 2007) was of 2.5 per 100,000 persons per year. U.S. incidence and mortality rates are about 2.5 and 2.8 in men and women, respectively.[12]

Generally, the highest HNSCC rates are found in Melanesia, South-Central Asia, and Central and Eastern Europe and the lowest in Africa, Central America, and Eastern Asia for both males and females.[13]

The incidence rates for HNSCC related to HPV infections, such as oropharynx, tonsil, and tongue base, are increasing in young adults in the United States and in some countries in Europe, which is hypothesized to be in part due to changes in oral sexual behavior.[14]

In this issue, the aim is to describe epigenetic mechanisms behind HNSCC. The main mechanisms evaluated are DNA methylation, posttranslational histone modification, and noncoding RNAs

2. Epigenetic mechanisms

2.1. DNA methylation

DNA methylation is a chemical marking system for annotating genetic information by causing gene repression through its ability to affect factor binding and chromatin structure.[14] This system has gene expression patterns that are regulated in a spatial and time-dependent manner.[5] Heritable information is carried by chemical modifications of both DNA and chromatin-associated proteins and modulates chromatin structure and DNA accessibility.[5]

DNA methylation refers to the methylation of DNA cytosine residues at the carbon 5 position.[15, 16] DNA methyltransferases (DNMTs) catalyze the transfer of a methyl group to position 5 of a cytosine, generating 5-methylcytosine (5mC).[17] This chemical modification affects gene expression when CpG-rich areas are present inside promoter regions (figure 3).[16, 18] This is accomplished by the activities of one or more DNA methyltransferases (DNMTs), which use S-adenosylmethionine (AdoMet) as a cofactor.[19]

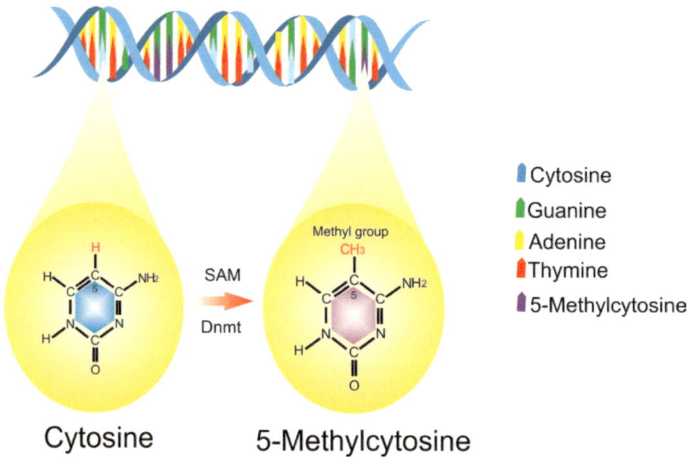

Figure 3. DNA methylation.

About 60% of human gene promoters are associated with CpG islands and are usually unmethylated in normal cells, although some of them (~6%) become methylated in a tissue-specific manner during early development or in differentiated tissues.[20]

Recent findings also suggest that extensive DNA methylation changes caused by differentiation take place at CpG island "shores," regions of comparatively low CpG density close to CpG islands.[2]

A relationship between DNA methylation and cancer has been found, given that DNA methyltransferases can be genetically altered in malignancies, that is, occur with DNMT3A20 and DNMT3B.[21] Aberrant DNA methylation is an epigenetic mechanism that contributes to the development of a wide variety of human cancers, either in the form of promoter-specific hypermethylation or genome-wide hypomethylation.[22] Hypermethylation in gene promoter regions is usually associated with expression suppression[23] and is the most common alterations in human cancers, leading to the abnormal expression of a broad spectrum of genes.[22] On the other hand, hypomethylation occurs in a large percentage in repetitive DNA elements.[24]

2.2. Posttranslational covalent histone modifications

Chromatin is the state in which DNA is packaged within the cell.[25] The chromatin architecture can be remodeled by a network of protein mediators called histones that play an important role in gene regulation by compacting DNA.[26] The nucleosome is the fundamental unit of chromatin, and it is composed of an octamer of histones (H2A, H2B, H3, and H4) around which 147 base pairs of DNA are wrapped.[25] Dynamic variations in the organization of chromatin structure are mediated by histone acetylation and deacetylation (figure 4).[25]

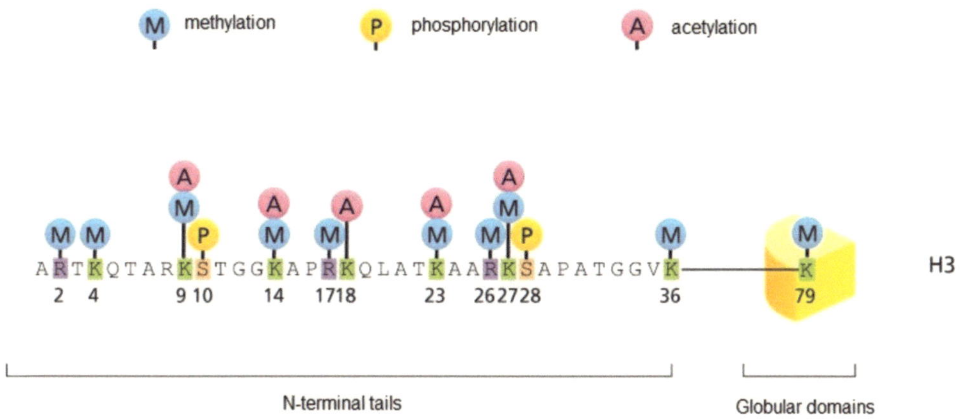

Figure 4. Posttranslational covalent histone modifications.

Acetylation neutralizes the positive charge of lysine residues, weakening charge-dependent interactions between histone and nucleosomal DNA, linker DNA, or adjacent histones, thus increasing the accessibility of DNA to the transcription machinery. Histone lysine acetylation also functions in other cellular processes that require DNA access.[27]

The posttranslational modification of histones by methylation is an important and widespread type of chromatin modification that is known to influence biological processes in the context of development and cellular responses.[28] Other modifications can be performed through lysine ubiquitination, serine phosphorylation, sumoylation, and methylation of lysines and arginines.[29]

Sumoylation is a process in which proteins are functionally or structurally similar to ubiquitin and are termed ubiquitin-like proteins (UBLs). UBLs include SUMO, NEDD8, ISG15, and FAT10.[30]

Histone acetyltransferases (HAT) catalyze the transfer of an acetyl group from acetyl-CoA to ε-amino group of a histone lysine residue.[31] The action of histone deacetylases (HDAC) is different because the effect is on the lysine residues. The first process involves chromatin decondensation, and the second process involves chromatin compaction. Either one or the other affects the gene transcription due to conformation changes in the chromatin.[31]

2.3. Noncoding RNAs

The noncoding RNAs are another level of epigenetic control for their capacity to establish other epigenetic marks and control gene expression.[4] Noncoding RNA (ncRNA) is a type of RNA that does not code for protein but has enzymatic, structural, or regulatory function.[32] ncRNAs can be classed as either small or long ncRNA, based on their transcript length.[33, 34]

2.4. MicroRNAs

MicroRNAs (miRNAs) are a set of non-protein-coding RNAs that bind to partially complementary sites in the 3′-untranslated regions of their messenger RNA targets.[35] MicroRNAs are the 21–23 nucleotide single-stranded RNA molecules found in eukaryotic cells.[36] The miRNAs interfere with messenger RNA translation or cause messenger RNA degradation, thereby repressing gene expression posttranscriptionally (Figure 5).[37] This is possible through imperfect base pairing with the 3′-untranslated region (3′-UTR) of target mRNAs of protein-coding genes, leading to the cleavage of homologous mRNA or translational inhibition.[38]

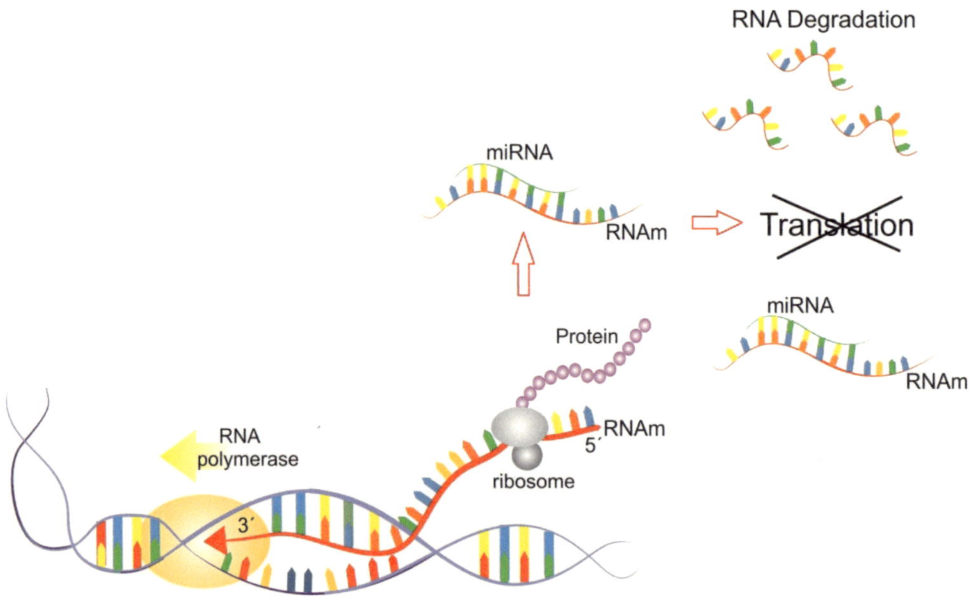

Figure 5. RNA degradation by miRNA.

miRNAs are transcribed for the most part by RNA polymerase II as long primary transcripts characterized by hairpin structures (pri-miRNA) and are processed in the nucleus by RNase III Drosha into 70–100 nucleotide long precursor miRNAs (pre-miRNAs).[39]

MicroRNAs are partial complementarity between their target transcripts. A single microRNA is capable of simultaneously regulating up to hundreds of genes, giving rise to an enormous modulatory potential.[40]

MicroRNAs are involved in a variety of cellular processes, including the regulation of cellular differentiation, proliferation, and apoptosis, and an aberrant expression of miRNA is known to induce various human malignancies.[41] New evidence suggests that miRNAs can act as

http://dx.doi.org/10.5772/61135

oncogenes or tumor suppressors, exerting a key function in tumorigenesis.[42] Recently, a new function mediating tumor metastasis in breast cancer has been assigned to miRNAs, by which this malignant step is promoted or suppressed.[42]

2.5. Long noncoding RNAs

Long noncoding RNAs (lncRNAs) are generated by the same transcriptional machinery as are other mRNAs. These lncRNAs have a 5′ terminal methylguanosine cap and are often spliced and polyadenylated.[45] lncRNAs have length greater than 200 nucleotides without protein-coding potential but with a wide range of structural and functional roles.[34] Some of this process can include the chromatin remodeling and transcriptional control assemblies.[31] They are generally transcriptionally activated or repressed by associated transcription factors and function as molecular mediators of gene expression.[43] When the lncRNAs act as molecular scaffolds, they can guide the chromatin-modifying complexes to bind into specific genomic loci. This way, they impart a repressive or activating effect on gene expression (Figure 6).[43]

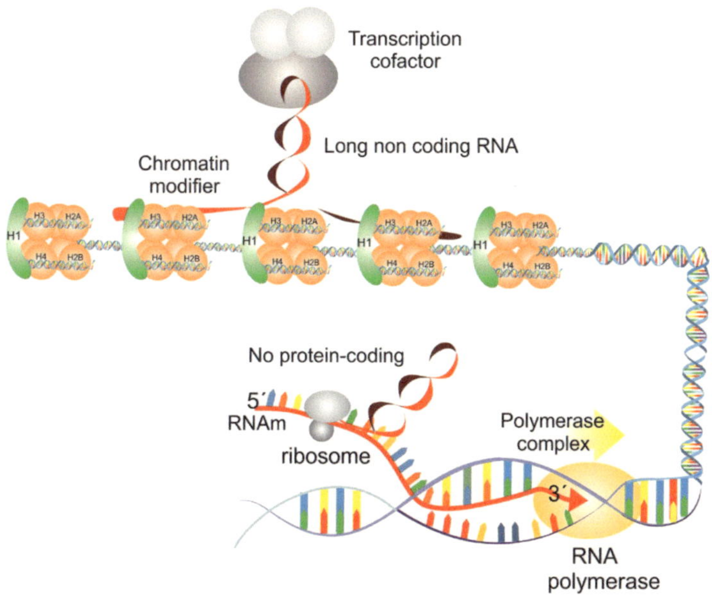

Figure 6. Long noncoding RNA.

According to their association with mRNA, the LncRNAs can be divided in different categories[44]: this can overlap with coding regions of a transcript on the same strand and with coding regions of a transcript on the opposite strand. This can be intronic lncRNAs from other transcript and can be intergenic lncRNAs between two genes on the same strand.[45]

The functions of the RNA in regulation of gene expression can be summarizing at transcriptional levels, RNA processing, and translation. Furthermore, they can protect genomes from foreign nucleic acids. At chromatin level, they can modulate the genome rearrangement.

Finally, the ncRNAs can operate as RNA–protein complexes, including ribosomes, snRNPs, snoRNPs, telomerase, microRNAs, and long ncRNAs.[46]

Long noncoding RNAs have also been shown to be necessary for targeting histone-modifying activities. Histone methylation is the end result of the transcription of long noncoding RNAs and the subsequent nucleation and targeting of histone modifying completes.[27]

The aberrant expression of lncRNAs has been associated with human cancers, suggesting a critical role in tumorigenesis.[47, 48] It has been demonstrated that a novel lncRNA, HOTAIR, was up-regulated and promoted cancer metastasis and predicted poor prognosis in ESCC.[34] Additionally, the association of dysregulated lncRNAs with specific developmental stages and clinical outcomes indicates their potential as strong diagnostic and prognostic predictors as well as therapeutic targets.[49]

3. Epigenetic changes in head and neck cancer

3.1. DNA methylation in head and neck cancer

The DNA methylation events in HNSCC include genes involved in cell cycle regulation, signal transduction, secreted protein, transmembrane protein, transcription factors, prostaglandin metabolism, metal ion homeostasis, oxidative stress, and oncoviruses.[50] Additionally, HNSCCs have genes involved in DNA damage repair, apoptosis, Wnt signaling, signal transduction, tissue invasion/metastasis, tumor suppression, and others (Figure 7, Table 1).[13, 51]

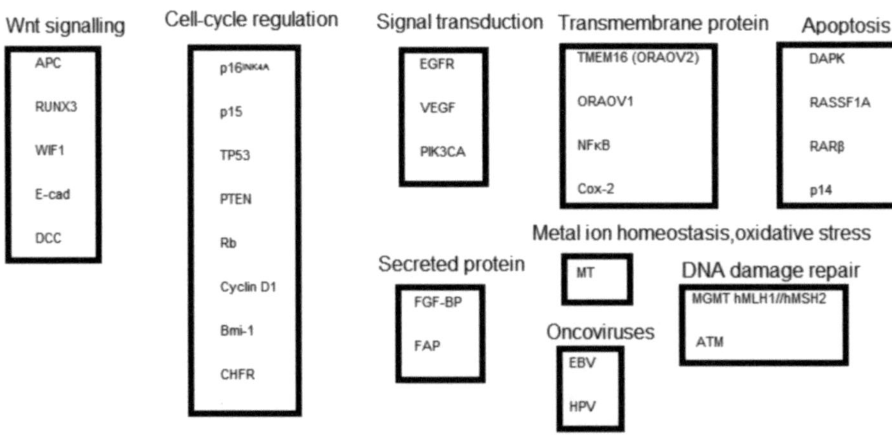

Figure 7. Genes and DNA methylation in HNSCC. Modified from Magić et al.,[13] Polanska et al.,[50] and Kaabi et al.[51]

http://dx.doi.org/10.5772/61135

Major classes	Member	Function
Cell cycle regulation	p16^{INK4A}	A tumor suppressor gene regulating senescence and cell cycle progression
	p15	Cyclin-dependent kinase inhibitor
	TP53	A tumor suppressor gene regulating cell cycle progression and cell survival
	PTEN	A tumor suppressor gene regulating signaling pathways controlling cell proliferation and apoptosis
	Rb	A proto-oncogene regulating cell cycle progression
	Cyclin D1	Controls cell cycle and self-renewal of tissue stem cells
	Bmi-1	Transmembrane TK that acts as a central transducer of multiple signaling pathways
	CHFR	Early G2/M checkpoint
Signal transduction	EGFR	A transmembrane TK that acts as a central transducer of multiple signaling pathways
	VEGF	A transmembrane TK that promotes proliferation, migration, and survival of endothelial cells during tumor growth
	PIK3CA	A gene encoding the p110a subunit of phosphoinositide 3-kinase (PI3K) α
Secreted protein	FGF-BP	Fibroblast growth factors binding protein
	FAP	Protein secreted by cancer-associated stroma
Transmembrane protein	TMEM16 (ORAOV2)	Calcium-activated chloride channel
	ORAOV1	A regulator of cell growth and tumor angiogenesis
	NFκB	Proinflammatory transcription factor
	Cox-2	Catalyzes prostaglandin synthesis from arachidonic acid
Metal ion homeostasis, oxidative stress	MT	Low molecular weight proteins involved in heavy metal detoxification, essential metal ion homeostasis, and cell protection against free radicals
Oncoviruses	EBV	A causative agent for most nasopharyngeal carcinomas, plasma EBV DNA load is an independent prognostic factor
	HPV	A causative agent for most oropharyngeal cancers
DNA damage repair	MGMT	DNA repair for alkylated guanine
	hMLH1//hMS	DNA mismatch repair
	H2 ATM	DNA double-strand breaks

Major classes	Member	Function
Apoptosis	DAPK	p53-dependent apoptosis
	RASSF1A	RAS pathway regulation and tumor suppression
	RARβ	Regulatory protein and apoptosis
	p14	Proapoptosis
Wnt signaling	APC	Wnt signaling and adhesion
	RUNX3	Wnt signaling inhibitor, TGF-β-induced tumor sup pression
	WIF1	Secreted Wnt antagonist
	E-cad	Cell adhesion, forming adherens junctions
	DCC	Cell–cell adhesion
Signal transduction	SFRP1	Antagonists of the Wnt pathway
	EDNRB	Endothelin receptor type B
	RUNX3	Wnt pathway antagonist
Tumor suppression	HIN1	Inhibitor Ras pathway
	DAPK1	Proapoptosis
	DCC	Proapoptosis
	RASSF1A/RASSF2	Negative RAS effector, proapoptotic, microtubule stabilization
Others	KIF1A	Cell division and microtubule-dependent intracellular organelle transport

Table 1. Genes and DNA methylation in HNSCC. Modified from Magić et al.,[13] Polanska et al.,[50] and Kaabi et al. [51]

The primary risk factors for the development of HNSCC include tobacco use, alcohol consumption, human papillomavirus (HPV) infections (mainly for oropharyngeal cancers), and Epstein–Barr virus (EBV) infections (for nasopharyngeal cancer).[52]

In promoter methylation, the p16 and p15 genes are commonly observed in human epithelial malignancies, including HNSCC. Histologically normal surgical margin epithelium of HNSCC patients with chronic smoking and drinking habits has a significantly higher prevalence of p15 methylation compared with nonsmokers and nondrinkers.[53]

Between genes that have been associated with hypermethylation, the p16 and the p14 genes undergo inactivation due to promoter hypermethylation.[13] Encoded by the CDKN2A gene, p16 inhibits cyclin-dependent kinases 4 and 6, thus blocking the promotion of cells from the G1 to the S phase of the cell cycle.[54] CDKN2A (p16) inactivation is common in lung cancer and occurs via homozygous deletions, methylation of promoter region, or point mutations.[55] CDKN2A (p16) disruption is reported as a frequent event in head and neck squamous cell carcinomas that confers poor prognosis.[56] Other genes as DAP-K, RASSF1A, RARß2, and MGMT have been reported as genes under hypermethylation promotor but with functions in DNA repair. These genes removed mutagenic (O6-guanine) adducts from DNA.[57]

DAPK and RASSF1A genes have shown methylation in HNSCC.[58] The methylation of p16 could be an initial process that might address abnormalities or deregulation of cell cycle controls.[59]

The ataxia-telangiectasia-mutated (*ATM*) gene produces a protein kinase that functions as a tumor suppressor by triggering appropriate cellular response to genome damage resulting from ionizing radiation or chemical carcinogen exposure.[60] It is currently unknown whether ATM is lost in HNSCCs displaying the deletion in the 11q22–23 locus.[61]

Aggressive HNSCC has been linked to expression loss of E-cadherin (ECAD) protein.[51] The protein ECAD can be inactivated by promoter hypermethylation.[62] In patients with HNSCC who are low smokers, the hypermethylation of CDH1 occurs more commonly, suggesting that an additional factor may be driving this epigenetic alteration.[62]

Cyclooxygenase-2 (Cox-2) is presumed to contribute to cancer progression through its multifaceted function, and recently its inverse relationship with E-cadherin was suggested. Increased expression of Cox-2 has been found in a variety of human malignancies, including HNSCC. [63]

The death-associated protein kinase (DAPk) family contains three closely related serine/ threonine kinases, namely, DAPk, ZIPk, and DRP-1, which display a high degree of homology in their catalytic domains.[64] The methylation profile of DAPK in HNSCC (including oral squamous cell carcinoma) is a promising biomarker for the follow-up and early detection of head and neck cancer recurrence.[65]

The Ras association domain family protein 1A (RASSF1A) is arguably one of the most frequently inactivated tumor suppressors in human cancer. RASSF1A modulates apoptosis via the Hippo and Bax pathways but also modulates the cell cycle.[66] The epigenetic inactivation of RASSF1A plays an important role in the development of cancer.[67]

TP53, once activated, leads to apoptosis and growth arrest (either cell cycle arrest or senescence). It is clear that TP53 mutation is common in HNSCC.[68] The p53 transcription factor stands out as a key tumor suppressor and a master regulator of various signaling pathways involved in this process.[69] Tobacco smoke is the best known and studied mutagen involved in lung carcinogenesis, and TP53 mutational patterns differ between smokers and nonsmokers, with an excess of G to T transversions in smoking-associated cancer.[69]

The Cancer Genome Atlas has informed about smoking-related HNSCCs and its relations with the universal loss of function of TP53 mutations and CDKN2A. This inactivation is accompanied with frequent copy number alterations, including amplification of 3q26/28 and 11q13/22.[70]

The phosphatidylinositol 3-kinase (PI3K)/AKT/mTOR pathway is antagonized by phosphatase and tensin homologue (PTEN). PTEN protein is a tumor suppressor frequently disrupted in cancer, altering tumor cell growth and survival.[71] The decrease in PTEN function in HNSCC is due to several genetic and epigenetic alterations. Recently, promoter hypermethylation has been implicated in the down-regulation of PTEN in HNSCC cell lines.[72]

HNSCCs also exhibit many chromosomal abnormalities, including amplifications of the 11q13 region containing the cyclin D1 gene and the 7p11 region encoding EGFR, which lead to proto-oncogene activation.[73] The most critical point in regulation of the cell cycle is the G1 checkpoint. Cyclin D1, a G1 cyclin, has been implicated in the regulation of the G1 to S phase progression in many different cell types. Cyclin D1 forms active complexes that promote the phosphorylation of retinoblastoma protein (RB) and the activation of E2F-responsive gene.[74]

PIK3CA is a human gene that regulates various cellular functions, including proliferation and invasion. Because it is an oncogene, its activation by either gene amplification or mutation results in a cellular growth advantage contributing toward cancer formation and progression.[75] Mutations in PIK3CA have cases displayed of concurrent amplification. Additionally, some tumors (20%) contain focal amplification without evidence of mutation. The largest mutation proportions of PIK3CA are localized to hotspots that promote activation.[70] PIK3CA is an active mutation that is common in conjunction with infrequent copy number alteration, and it forms part of a subgroup of oral cavity tumors with favorable clinical outcomes.[70]

Bmi1 (B-cell-specific Moloney Murine Leukemia virus insertion site 1) is a transcription repressor for cell senescence, implicated in the self-renewal of stem cell. Bmi1 is highly expressed in the CD44+ cell population sorted from oral SCC tumors.[76]

E3 ubiquitin-protein ligase (CHFR) is a gene involved in a checkpoint regulating entry to mitosis.[77] Loss of CHFR leads to mitotic catastrophe and apoptosis due to mitotic spindle alteration. Aberrant methylation of the gene has been reported in several primary tumor genes. EGFR is a potential prognostic biomarker.[78]

Epidermal growth factor receptor (erb-B1) is a member of the erbB family of tyrosine kinase receptor proteins.[79] Previous studies have shown that EGFR is expressed or highly expressed in various human tumor cells.[79] The overexpression of EGFR is attributed to gene amplification, which is noted to be about 12 copies per cell in relation to head and neck squamous cell carcinomas. The constitutive EGFR activation caused via autocrine stimulation and through the coexpression of EGFR with its ligands, TGFα, has been observed and is indicative of its poor prognosis.[72] EGFR-targeted therapy is commonly used for the treatment of advanced HNSCC due to numerous findings that describe overexpression and/or high activity of EGFR in the majority of HNSCC.[80]

Various factors are known to regulate angiogenesis; for example, vascular endothelial cell growth factor (VEGF) has potent angiogenic effects. The presence of VEGF has been reported in approximately 40% of head and neck squamous cell carcinomas (HNSCCs), and its presence is associated with a poor prognosis.[72]

Other mechanisms included in the tumorous angiogenesis lie in the intake and utilization of locally stored fibroblast growth factors (FGFs).[50] FGF-1 (aFGF) and FGF-2 (bFGF) are found in most embryonic and adult normal and tumor tissues, where they are immobilized in the extracellular matrix (ECM).[81]

Fibroblast activation protein (FAP) is a member of the serine protease family that is selectively expressed in the stromal fibroblasts associated with epithelial cancers and is expressed at low or undetectable levels in the resting fibroblasts of normal adult tissues. FAP is expressed in more than 90% of epithelial carcinomas, which makes it a promising target.[82]

Oral cancer overexpressed 1 and 2 (ORAOV1-ORAOV2) overexpression was reported in HNSCC.[50, 83] The first is required for cell growth and tumor angiogenesis,[84] and the second is required in the modulation of TMEM16A activity in various epithelial tissues.[85]

Multiple signaling pathways have been linked to tumor resistance, including activation of nuclear factor kappa B (NFκB).[86] NFκB is an epigenetic modifier that plays a major role in malignant transformation, and this pathway serves as a target for epigenetic drugs.[26] The constitutive activation of NFκB signaling is often observed in HNSCC, suggesting a common epigenetic mechanism in HNSCC biology. Indeed, the activation of NFκB signaling in HNSCC induced chromatin compaction and acquisition of resistance to chemotherapy.[26]

Metallothionein (MT) is a family of cysteine-rich, low molecular weight (500–14,000 Da) proteins. MTs have been proposed to play important roles in protecting against DNA damage, apoptosis, and oxidative stress. MT is a tumor suppressor reported to show promoter hypermethylated in various cancers.[87]

Human mismatch repair genes (hMMR) have the ability to repair both mismatched bases and insertion loop errors during DNA replication.[88] Suboptimal DNA repair could result in disrupting the pattern of repeat sequences, causing chromosomal aberrations in the genome of patients suffering from instability syndromes. Significant proportions of carcinomas develop through DNA mismatch repair genes (MMR) deficiency and exhibit frequent microsatellite alteration (MA).[88]

The hypermethylated adenomatosis polyposis coli (APC) tumor suppressor gene has reduced expression levels along with loss of heterozygosity (LOH), leading to the altered functioning of the APC tumor suppressor proteins, which play a role for the integrity and function of the β-catenin destruction complex.[72] The APC protein, a negative regulator of this pathway, has been strongly implicated in the development of colon cancer but still has an undetermined role in the formation of oral cancer.[89]

Loss of heterozygosity of the APC gene and epigenetic events lead to the decreased expression of APC and the Wnt antagonists, the secreted frizzled-related proteins (SFRPs), Wnt inhibitory factors (WIFs), and Dickkopf family members (DKKs), primarily by promoter hypermethylation.[90] The persistent β-catenin signaling contributes to increased growth, metastatic potential, and resistance to chemotherapy in HNSCC and their tumor-initiating cells.[90] The methylation of WIF-1 correlated with shorter survival in oral cancer patients. The methylation of WIF1 may be considered a prognostic marker in oral cancers.[91]

Wnt pathway stimulates several intracellular signal transduction cascades (canonical and noncanonical).[92] The possible role of RUNX3 as a tumor suppressor in HNSCC has been reported. The promoter hypermethylation of antagonist's genes to Wnt (RUNX3) has been identified as a common event in cancer.[93]

Deleted in colorectal cancer (DCC) is a candidate tumor suppressor gene located at chromosome 18q21.[94] DCC promoter region hypermethylation was found in 75% of primary HNSCC. There was a significant correlation between DCC promoter region hypermethylation and DCC expression.[94] DCC is a putative conditional tumor suppressor gene that is epigenetically inactivated by promoter hypermethylation in a majority of HNSCC.[94, 95]

Secreted frizzled-related protein (SFRP1) is epigenetically silenced and functions as a tumor suppressor in oral squamous cell carcinoma (OSCC). The loss of SFRP2 expression is associated with hypermethylation of its promoter.[96]

The methylation of the *KIF1A* and *EDNRB* gene promoters is a frequent event in HNSCC.[97] KIF1A (kinesin family member 1A) encodes a protein that is a microtubule-dependent molecular motor involved in important intracellular functions such as organelle transport and cell division.[98] Endothelin receptor type B (EDNRB) is a G-protein-coupled receptor that activates a phosphatidylinositol calcium second messenger system.[97, 99]

Runt domain transcription factors (RUNXs) are homologous to products encoded by the Drosophila segmentation genes runt and lozenge.[100] The *RUNX3* gene is located on human chromosome 1p36, a region that has long been suspected to harbor one or more suppressors of various tumors.[101] Inactivation of RUNX3, which is caused mainly by epigenetic alteration, is closely associated with bladder tumor development, recurrence, and progression.[100, 101]

HIN-1 (high in normal-1) is a putative cytokine with growth inhibitory activities and is down-regulated by aberrant methylation in breast cancers.[102] Evidence suggests that HIN-1 is a potential tumor suppressor gene in non-small cell lung cancer (NSCLC), silenced by promoter hypermethylation and negatively regulated by AKT signaling pathway.[103] Silencing of HIN-1 expression and methylation of its promoter occurs in multiple human cancer types, suggesting that the elimination of HIN-1 function may contribute to several forms of epithelial tumorigenesis.[104]

3.2. Histone modifications in head and neck cancer

Aberrant regulation of the demethylases controlling H3K9me3 and H4K20me3 levels could contribute to the oncogenic potential. For instance, levels of H3K4me2 and me3 are significantly different in oral squamous cell carcinoma in comparison with cells of the healthy tissues; the level of H3K4me2 is increased while that of H3K4me3 is decreased.[102, 105]

A similar trend was observed in tongue squamous cell carcinoma (SCC) cells where the levels of the H3K27me3 marks at chromatin near homeobox genes were inversely correlated with the transcript levels in nontumorigenic, immortalized human oral keratinocytes (OKF6-TERT1R) and tumorigenic oral SCC-9 cells.[25] This investigation found that the levels of the H3K27me3 marks at chromatin near homeobox genes were inversely correlated with the transcript levels in nontumorigenic, immortalized human oral keratinocytes (OKF6- TERT1R) and tumorigenic oral SCC-9 cells.[25]

The emerging importance of the regulation of the H3K27me3 mark as a driver of squamous differentiation suggests that SCCs may harbor defects in the epigenetic regulation of squamous differentiation.[106] The dysregulation of squamous differentiation is fundamental to the development of SCC and has been reported to occur early in premalignant lesions.[107]

On the other hand, serine phosphorylation plays an important role in assembling the DNA damage response complex by identifying DNA double-strand breaks (DSB) in the chromatin. Upon DSB, ATM induces the phosphorylation of γH2AX at serine 139, resulting in the recruitment of BRCA1, BRCA2, Rad51, Mre11, NBS1, FANCD2, and p53 repair proteins to sites of DNA damage.[108]

In addition, the phosphorylation of serine 536 involved in the phosphorylation of RELA has also been reported. RELA, also known as p65, is an REL-associated protein involved in NF-κB heterodimer formation, nuclear translocation, and activation.[109] The phosphorylation of serine 468 is also associated with RELA.[109]

Regarding sumoylation, there are also desumoylating enzymes called SENPs, which remove the SUMO residues from the sumoylated proteins. Two molecules involved in the SUMO pathway, Ubc9 and SENP5, are up-regulated in SCCs. The up-regulation of SENP5 is found in oral SCCs, and strong SENP5 expression is correlated with poor prognosis.[110]

Finally, the lysine methylation of HSP90AB1 is important for its homodimerization and its interaction with stress-induced phosphoprotein 1 (STIP1) and cell division cycle 37 (CDC37), which are co-chaperones of HSP90AB1 in human cancer cells, resulting in enhancement of cancer cell growth.[111]

3.3. miRNAs in head and neck cancer

DNA copy number variations or deregulation of miRNA expression has been shown to contribute to carcinogenesis, including carcinogenesis of HNSCC.[112] Several studies have reported global miRNA expression changes in carcinogenesis of HNSCC, using various samples sizes, anatomical sites, and profiling methodologies.[113]

It has been demonstrated the differential expression patterns of miRNAs in numerous types of cancer. MiR-92a, miR-103/107, miR-21, miR143, miR145, miR-205 and miR-296, among others, have been confirmed to be involved in the development of esophageal squamous cell carcinoma (ESCC).[34]

It has been reported that members of the miR-17-92 cluster were deregulated in 15 patients with OSCC (tongue and floor of the mouth) and 35 patients with HNSCC. The miR-19a and the miR-19b were strongly up-regulated. The miR-17-3p/miR-17-5p and the miR-92b were moderately up-regulated. Evidence has been found that the miR-17-92 cluster is up-regulated in many cancer types.[114] Furthermore, the miR-196a and the miR-10b, not previously associated with HNSCC, may play an oncogenic role in this disease through the deregulation of cell proliferation.[114]

Other studies informed that miR-21, miR-31, miR-504, and miR-10b are target tumor suppressor genes. These miRNAs are involved in HNSCC.[115] Many studies have confirmed the tumor suppressor roles of the let-7 family (the miR-99 family, miR-107, miR-133a, miR-137, miR-138, and miR-375). Other miRNAs such as miR-21, let-7, miR-107, miR-138, and miR-200c are involved in regulating stemness or the epithelial–mesenchymal transition of tumor cells.[115]

It has also been evaluated that miR-34a is significantly down-regulated in HNSCC tumors and cell lines.[116] The ectopic expression of miR-34a in HNSCC cell lines significantly inhibited tumor cell proliferation, colony formation, and migration. Tumor samples from HNSCC patients showed an inverse relationship between miR-34a and survival as well as between miR-34a and E2F3 levels.[116]

In silico analysis identified three putative microRNA-107 (miR-107) binding sites in the 3′-untranslated region (UTR) of PKCε.[117] An inverse relationship was revealed between miR-107 and PKCε in HNSCC cell lines. These data demonstrated that PKCε is directly regulated by miR-107 and, moreover, suggest that miR-107 may be a potential anticancer therapeutic for HNSCC.[117]

New computational approach strategies complementary to microRNA profiling are capable of simultaneously predicting tumor suppressor microRNAs as well as their functional targets from gene expression.[118] It provided a plausible mechanism that loss of the tumor suppressor function of miR-204 as a result of allelic imbalance at 9q21.1–q22.3 may significantly increase genetic susceptibility to HNSCC oncogenesis and progression.[118] The complete suppression of miR-204 and its host gene TRPM3 has become possible that the mRNA expression may serve as a marker the expression status in HNSCC.[118]

3.4. lncRNAs in head and neck cancer

LncRNAs have been linked to essential growth-promoting activities, and their deregulation contributes to tumor cell survival. A prominent example is the Hox transcript antisense intergenic lncRNA, HOTAIR.[119] The HOTAIR gene controls gene expression, and its expression is deregulated in a spectrum of cancers. Furthermore, HOTAIR expression correlates with patient survival.[119, 120]

HOTAIR serves as a scaffold for at least two distinct histone modification complexes. A 5′ domain of HOTAIR binds Polycomb Repressive Complex 2 (PRC2), while a 3′ domain of HOTAIR binds the LSD1/CoREST/REST complex. lncRNAPCAT-1, a target gene of polycomb repressive complex 2, has been implicated in disease progression by promoting cell proliferation.[121] The ability to link two distinct complexes enables RNA-mediated assembly of PRC2 and LSD1 and coordinates targeting of PRC2 and LSD1 to chromatin for coupled histone H3 lysine 27 methylation and lysine 4 demethylation.[122]

In prostate cancer, the up-regulation of antisense noncoding RNA in the INK4 locus (ANRIL) is required for the expression of the tumor suppressors INK4a/p16 and INK4b/p15.[121]

Some examples of lncRNAs that has a role in chromatin remolding include *XIST*, which acts by recruiting the PRC2 complex to initiate X-chromosome inactivation as well as *MALAT* and *NEAT1*, both of which play a role in mRNA processing and nuclear organization.[123]

The expression of LINC00312 in nasopharyngeal carcinoma has a tumor-suppressive function. Under physiological conditions, LINC00312 inhibits proliferation in nasopharyngeal epithelium by preventing cell cycle passage from the G1 into S phase but increases cell adhesion, motility, and invasion by down-regulating the expression of estrogen receptor alpha (ERα). [124]

Other genes regulated by lncRNAs that have been implicated in cancer include NDM29, BACE1AS, and Drosophila hsr-ω gene.[125] Neuroblastoma differentiation Marker 29 (NDM29) is an RNA polymerase (pol) III-transcribed noncoding (nc) RNA whose synthesis drives neuroblastoma (NB) cell differentiation to a nonmalignant neuron-like phenotype.[126] BACE1 plays a pivotal role in the accumulation of β-amyloid plaques and has been shown to regulate the expression of BACE1 by increasing BACE1 mRNA stability.[127] The heat shock RNA omega (hsrω) gene of *Drosophila melanogaster* is inducible by cell stress and provides structural base for sequestering diverse RNA-processing/regulatory proteins.[128]

4. Clinical applications in head and neck cancer

To date, four epigenetic inhibitors have been approved by the U.S. Food and Drug Administration (FDA) for cancer treatment.[129] The DNMT inhibitors as 5-aza-cytidine and 5-aza-2′-deoxycytidine are widely used in in vitro in research. The cytosine analogs are converted to deoxynucleotide triphosphates inside the cell and then incorporated into the DNA during replication in the original C positions.[130]

Other inhibitors of HATs approved by FDA are p300, lysine methyltransferases (H3K79 methyltransferase DOT1L, or the polycomb complex member EZH2), and lysine demethylases (LSd1). Furthermore, small molecule inhibitors targeting the histone reader, BRD4, have also shown promise as therapeutic agent in many cancer types.[131]

The effects of an epigenetic inhibitor as lysine residues on histone tails are HDAC inhibitors that counteract the global overexpression of HDACs in cancer and reinstate a more permissive nucleosome structure for transcription.[132] Vorinostat (a pan-HDAC inhibitor) and romidepsin (a class I HDAC inhibitor) have each shown >30% response rates against cutaneous T-cell lymphoma (CTCL) in phase II trials.[132]

Cetuximab is an inhibitor of the epidermal growth factor receptor (EGFR) that is used in radiation therapy. It was found to enhance HNSCC patient survival compared with radiation therapy alone.[133] The FDA has approved cetuximab to treat HNSCC; the drug has a response rate of about 10% when used as a single agent in recurrent/metastatic disease.[134] However, despite approval of cetuximab, improvement in patient survival with the use of this agent has been only modestly incremental.[133]

Advances in oncogenomics have also identified mutations in epigenetic-associated genes that encode histones and their linkers, proteins associated with the recruitment of DNA-binding proteins, HDAC I and II interacting proteins, corepressor proteins, and transcriptional activators and coactivators.[135]

The understanding of which gene mutations, DNA methylation, posttranslational histone modification, and noncoding RNAs drive the carcinogenesis may help us understand how tumor susceptibility guides the development of new combination therapies. However, it is important remember that not all cancers are equally susceptible to epigenetic therapies. The biology underpinning this observation urgently warrants our attention if epigenetic therapies are to be more widely applicable.[136]

5. Conclusions

Understanding the complexity of the epigenome, the different dynamics, and the different subunits is complex and intimidating. Gene mutations, DNA methylation, posttranslational histone modification, and noncoding RNAs are actors involved in modulating its interactions with genomic sequences, and this is fundamental for health and disease.

Only our hope and desire can continue creating new ways to interact with the epigenome, and it will be possible to build a new world where the HNSCC and other types of cancer will be able to have new therapies and new opportunities for a better life.

Author details

Julio Cesar Osorio[1] and Andres Castillo[2*]

*Address all correspondence to: acastillo.doc@gmail.com

1 School of Biomedical Sciences, Universidad del Valle, Cali, Colombia

2 Biology Department, Faculty of Exact and Natural Sciences of Universidad del Valle, Cali, Colombia

References

[1] Gibney ER, Nolan CM. Epigenetics and gene expression. Heredity. 2010 07//print; 105(1):4–13.

[2] Rodriguez-Paredes M, Esteller M. Nature Medicine. 2011;17(null):330.

[3] Bernstein BE, Stamatoyannopoulos JA, Costello JF, Ren B, Milosavljevic A, Meissner A, et al. The NIH roadmap epigenomics mapping consortium. Nat Biotechnol. 2010 Oct;28(10):1045–8.

[4] Esteller M. Cancer epigenetics for the 21st century: what's next? Genes and Cancer. 2011 Jun;2(6):604–6.

[5] Park YJ, Claus R, Weichenhan D, Plass C. Genome-wide epigenetic modifications in cancer. Progress in Drug Research. 2011;67:25–49.

[6] Ragin CC, Taioli E. Survival of squamous cell carcinoma of the head and neck in relation to human papillomavirus infection: review and meta-analysis. International Journal of Cancer. 2007 Oct 15;121(8):1813–20.

[7] Magić Z, Supić G, Branković-Magić M, Jović N. DNA Methylation in the Pathogenesis of Head and Neck Cancer. 2012 2012-11-28.

[8] Mao L, Hong WK, Papadimitrakopoulou VA. Focus on head and neck cancer. Cancer Cell. 5(4):311–6.

[9] Harrison LB, Sessions RB, Hong WK. Head and Neck Cancer: A Multidisciplinary Approach. Lipppincott Williams & Wilkins; 2009.

[10] Koffler J, Sharma S, Hess J. Predictive value of epigenetic alterations in head and neck squamous cell carcinoma. Molecular and Cellular Oncology. 2014 2014/06/16;1(2):e954827.

[11] American Cancer Society. Cancer Facts & Figures 2014. Atlanta: American Cancer Society; 2014.

[12] Ferlay J, Shin HR, Bray F, Forman D, Mathers C, Parkin DM. Estimates of worldwide burden of cancer in 2008: GLOBOCAN 2008. International journal of cancer. 2010;127(12):2893–917.

[13] Jemal A, Bray F, Center MM, Ferlay J, Ward E, Forman D. Global cancer statistics. CA Cancer J Clin. 2011 Mar–Apr;61(2):69–90.

[14] Bergman Y, Cedar H. DNA methylation dynamics in health and disease. Nature Structural and Molecular Biology. 2013;20(3):274–81.

[15] O'Sullivan E, Goggins M. DNA methylation analysis in human cancer. Methods in Molecular Biology. 2013;980:131–156.

[16] Herman JG, Graff JR, Myöhänen S, Nelkin BD, Baylin SB. Methylation-specific PCR: a novel PCR assay for methylation status of CpG islands. Proceedings of the National Academy of Sciences of the United States of America. 1996;93(18):9821–6.

[17] Witte T, Plass C, Gerhauser C. Pan-cancer patterns of DNA methylation. Genome Medicine. 2014;6(8):66.

[18] Dantas Machado AC, Zhou T, Rao S, et al. Evolving insights on how cytosine methylation affects protein–DNA binding. Briefings in Functional Genomics. 2015;14(1):61–73.

[19] Weisenberger DJ, Campan M, Long TI, Kim M, Woods C, Fiala E, et al. Analysis of repetitive element DNA methylation by MethyLight. Nucleic Acids Research. 2005;33(21):6823–36.

[20] Portela A, Esteller M. Epigenetic modifications and human disease. Nature Biotechnology. 2010;28(10):1057–68.

[21] Fernandez AF, Assenov Y, Martin-Subero JI, Balint B, Siebert R, Taniguchi H, et al. A DNA methylation fingerprint of 1628 human samples. Genome Research. 2012;22(2): 407–19.

[22] Lima SC, Hernandez-Vargas H, Simao T, Durand G, Kruel CD, Le Calvez-Kelm F, et al. Identification of a DNA methylome signature of esophageal squamous cell carcinoma and potential epigenetic biomarkers. Epigenetics. 2011 Oct 1;6(10):1217–27.

[23] Adorján P, Distler J, Lipscher E, Model F, Müller J, Pelet C, et al. Tumour class prediction and discovery by microarray-based DNA methylation analysis. Nucleic Acids Research. 2002 Mar 1, 2002;30(5):e21.

[24] Richards KL, Zhang B, Baggerly KA, Colella S, Lang JC, Schuller DE, et al. Genome-wide hypomethylation in head and neck cancer is more pronounced in HPV-negative tumors and is associated with genomic instability. PloS One. 2009;4(3):e4941.

[25] Marcinkiewicz KM, Gudas LJ. Altered histone mark deposition and DNA methylation at homeobox genes in human oral squamous cell carcinoma cells. Journal of Cellular Physiology. 2014;229(10):1405–16.

[26] Le JM, Squarize CH, Castilho RM. Histone modifications: targeting head and neck cancer stem cells. World Journal of Stem Cells. 2014 11/26;6(5):511–25. PubMed PMID: PMC4178252.

[27] Zentner GE, Henikoff S. Regulation of nucleosome dynamics by histone modifications. Nature Structural and Molecular Biology. 2013;20(3):259–66.

[28] Greer EL, Shi Y. Histone methylation: a dynamic mark in health, disease and inheritance. Nature Reviews. Genetics. 2012;13(5):343–57.

[29] Spotswood HT, Turner BM. An increasingly complex code. Journal of Clinical Investigation. 2002 Sep;110(5):577–82.

[30] Welchman RL, Gordon C, Mayer RJ. Ubiquitin and ubiquitin-like proteins as multifunctional signals. Nature Reviews. Molecular Cell Biology. 2005 Aug;6(8):599–609.

[31] Giudice FS, Pinto DS, Nör JE, Squarize CH, Castilho RM. Inhibition of histone deacetylase impacts cancer stem cells and induces epithelial-mesenchyme transition of head and neck cancer. PloS One. 2013 03/20;8(3):e58672.

[32] Kugel JF, Goodrich JA. Non-coding RNAs: key regulators of mammalian transcription. Trends in Biochemical Sciences. 2012 Apr;37(4):144–51.

[33] Costa FF. Non-coding RNAs: meet thy masters. Bioessays. 2010 Jul;32(7):599–608.

[34] Li SQ, Li F, Xiao Y, Wang CM, Tuo L, Hu J, et al. Comparison of long noncoding RNAs, microRNAs and messenger RNAs involved in initiation and progression of esophageal squamous cell carcinoma. Molecular Medicine Reports. 2014 Aug;10(2): 652–62.

[35] Schickel R, Boyerinas B, Park SM, Peter ME. MicroRNAs: key players in the immune system, differentiation, tumorigenesis and cell death. Oncogene. 2008 Oct 6;27(45): 5959–74.

[36] Zhou X, Yang PC. MicroRNA: a small molecule with a big biological impact. MicroRNA (Shariqah, United Arab Emirates). 2012;1(1):1.

[37] Avissar M, McClean MD, Kelsey KT, Marsit CJ. MicroRNA expression in head and neck cancer associates with alcohol consumption and survival. Carcinogenesis. 2009 Dec 1, 2009;30(12):2059–63.

[38] Shiiba M, Uzawa K, Tanzawa H. MicroRNAs in head and neck squamous cell carcinoma (HNSCC) and oral squamous cell carcinoma (OSCC). Cancers. 2010;2(2):653–69.

[39] Takahashi R-u, Miyazaki H, Ochiya T. The role of microRNAs in the regulation of cancer stem cells. Frontiers in Genetics. 2013;4:295.

[40] Avissar M, Christensen BC, Kelsey KT, Marsit CJ. MicroRNA expression ratio is predictive of head and neck squamous cell carcinoma. Clinical Cancer Research. 2009;15(8):2850–5.

[41] Kimura S, Naganuma S, Susuki D, Hirono Y, Yamaguchi A, Fujieda S, et al. Expression of microRNAs in squamous cell carcinoma of human head and neck and the esophagus: miR-205 and miR-21 are specific markers for HNSCC and ESCC. Oncology Reports. 2010 Jun;23(6):1625–33.

[42] Lujambio A, Calin GA, Villanueva A, Ropero S, Sánchez-Céspedes M, Blanco D, et al. A microRNA DNA methylation signature for human cancer metastasis. Proceedings of the National Academy of Sciences. 2008 Sept 9, 2008;105(36):13556–61.

[43] Ghosal S, Das S, Chakrabarti J. Long noncoding RNAs: new players in the molecular mechanism for maintenance and differentiation of pluripotent stem cells. Stem Cells and Development. 2013 Aug 15;22(16):2240–53.

[44] Quan M, Chen J, Zhang D. Exploring the secrets of long noncoding RNAs. Pichler M, editor. International Journal of Molecular Sciences. 2015;16(3):5467–5496.

[45] Mercer TR, Mattick JS. Structure and function of long noncoding RNAs in epigenetic regulation. Nature Structural and Molecular Biology. 2013;20(3):300–7.

[46] Cech Thomas R, Steitz Joan A. The noncoding RNA revolution—trashing old rules to forge new ones. Cell.157(1):77–94.

[47] Gibb EA, Enfield KS, Stewart GL, Lonergan KM, Chari R, Ng RT, et al. Long non-coding RNAs are expressed in oral mucosa and altered in oral premalignant lesions. Oral Oncology. 2011 Nov;47(11):1055–61.

[48] Qi P, Du X. The long non-coding RNAs, a new cancer diagnostic and therapeutic gold mine. Modern Pathology. 2013;26(2):155–65.

[49] Xu M-d, Qi P, Du X. Long non-coding RNAs in colorectal cancer: implications for pathogenesis and clinical application. Modern Pathology. 2014;27(10):1310–20.

[50] Polanska H, Raudenska M, Gumulec J, Sztalmachova M, Adam V, Kizek R, et al. Clinical significance of head and neck squamous cell cancer biomarkers. Oral Oncology. 2014;50(3):168–77.

[51] Al-Kaabi A, van Bockel LW, Pothen AJ, Willems SM. p16INK4A and p14ARF gene promoter hypermethylation as prognostic biomarker in oral and oropharyngeal squamous cell carcinoma: a review. Disease Markers. 2014;2014:8.

[52] Ovchinnikov DA, Wan Y, Coman WB, Pandit P, Cooper-White JJ, Herman JG, et al. DNA methylation at the novel CpG sites in the promoter of MED15/PCQAP gene as a biomarker for head and neck cancers. Biomarker Insights. 2014;9:53–60.

[53] Wong TS, Man MW, Lam AK, Wei WI, Kwong YL, Yuen AP. The study of p16 and p15 gene methylation in head and neck squamous cell carcinoma and their quantitative evaluation in plasma by real-time PCR. European Journal of Cancer. 2003 Sept; 39(13):1881–7.

[54] Pierini S, Jordanov SH, Mitkova AV, Chalakov IJ, Melnicharov MB, Kunev KV, et al. Promoter hypermethylation of CDKN2A, MGMT, MLH1, and DAPK genes in laryngeal squamous cell carcinoma and their associations with clinical profiles of the patients. Head and Neck. 2014;36(8):1103–8.

[55] Tam KW, Zhang W, Soh J, Stastny V, Chen M, Sun H, et al. CDKN2A/p16 inactivation mechanisms and their relationship to smoke exposure and molecular features in non-small-cell lung cancer. Journal of Thoracic Oncology. 2013 Nov;8(11):1378–88.

[56] Lim AM, Do H, Young RJ, Wong SQ, Angel C, Collins M, et al. Differential mechanisms of CDKN2A (p16) alteration in oral tongue squamous cell carcinomas and correlation with patient outcome. International Journal of Cancer. 2014;135(4):887–95.

[57] Worsham MJ, Stephen JK, Chen KM, Havard S, Shah V, Gardner G, et al. Delineating an epigenetic continuum in head and neck cancer. Cancer Letters. 2014 Jan 28;342(2): 178–84.

[58] Supic G, Kozomara R, Brankovic-Magic M, Jovic N, Magic Z. Gene hypermethylation in tumor tissue of advanced oral squamous cell carcinoma patients. Oral Oncology. 2009 Dec;45(12):1051–7.

[59] Laytragoon-Lewin N, Chen F, Castro J, Elmberger G, Rutqvist LE, Lewin F, et al. DNA content and methylation of p16, DAPK and RASSF1A Gene in tumour and dis-

tant, normal mucosal tissue of head and neck squamous cell carcinoma patients. Anticancer Research. 2010 Nov 1, 2010;30(11):4643–8.

[60] Ai L, Vo QN, Zuo C, Li L, Ling W, Suen JY, et al. Ataxia-telangiectasia-mutated (ATM) gene in head and neck squamous cell carcinoma: promoter hypermethylation with clinical correlation in 100 cases. Cancer Epidemiology Biomarkers and Prevention. 2004 Jan 1, 2004;13(1):150–6.

[61] Chen Y, Chen C. DNA copy number variation and loss of heterozygosity in relation to recurrence of and survival from head and neck squamous cell carcinoma: a review. Head and Neck. 2008 Oct;30(10):1361–83.

[62] Marsit CJ, Posner MR, McClean MD, Kelsey KT. Hypermethylation of E-cadherin is an independent predictor of improved survival in head and neck squamous cell carcinoma. Cancer. 2008 Oct 1;113(7):1566–71.

[63] Fujii R, Imanishi Y, Shibata K, Sakai N, Sakamoto K, Shigetomi S, et al. Restoration of E-cadherin expression by selective Cox-2 inhibition and the clinical relevance of the epithelial-to-mesenchymal transition in head and neck squamous cell carcinoma. Journal of Experimental and Clinical Cancer Research. 2014;33(1):40.

[64] Gozuacik D, Kimchi A. DAPk protein family and cancer. Autophagy. 2006 Apr–Jun; 2(2):74–9.

[65] Liu M, Feng L, Tang X, Guo X. Gene promoter hypermethylation in leukoplakia of the oral mucosa. Pathology and Laboratory Medicine International. 2010;2:71–7.

[66] Donninger H, Clark JA, Monaghan MK, Schmidt ML, Vos M, Clark GJ. Cell cycle restriction is more important than apoptosis induction for RASSF1A protein tumor suppression. Journal of Biological Chemistry. 2014 Nov 7;289(45):31287–95.

[67] Koutsimpelas D, Pongsapich W, Heinrich ULF, Mann S, Mann WJ, Brieger J. Promoter methylation of MGMT, MLH1 and RASSF1A tumor suppressor genes in head and neck squamous cell carcinoma: pharmacological genome demethylation reduces proliferation of head and neck squamous carcinoma cells. Oncology Reports. 2012;27(4): 1135–41.

[68] Mitra S, Mukherjee N, Das S, Das P, Panda CK, Chakrabarti J. Anomalous altered expressions of downstream gene-targets in TP53-miRNA pathways in head and neck cancer. Scientific Reports. 2014 09/04/online;4.

[69] Rivlin N, Brosh R, Oren M, Rotter V. Mutations in the p53 tumor suppressor gene: important milestones at the various steps of tumorigenesis. Genes and Cancer. 2011;2(4):466–74.

[70] The Cancer Genome Atlas N. Comprehensive genomic characterization of head and neck squamous cell carcinomas. Nature. 2015;517(7536):576–82.

[71] M. Dillon L, W. Miller T. Therapeutic targeting of cancers with loss of PTEN function. Current Drug Targets. 2014 //;15(1):65–79.

[72] Grover J, Rakheja M, Rao NN, Singh A, Solomon MC. Emerging strategies against head and neck cancer—a review. IOSR Journal of Dental and Medical Sciences. 2014;13(9):138–47.

[73] Guerrero-Preston R, Michailidi C, Marchionni L, Pickering CR, Frederick MJ, Myers JN, et al. Key tumor suppressor genes inactivated by "greater promoter" methylation and somatic mutations in head and neck cancer. Epigenetics. 2014;9(7):1031–46.

[74] Iizuka S, Oridate N, Nashimoto M, Fukuda S, Tamura M. Growth Inhibition of head and neck squamous cell carcinoma cells by sgRNA targeting the cyclin D1 mRNA based on TRUE gene silencing. PloS One. 2014;9(12):e114121.

[75] Park B. PIK3CA Oncogene. In: Schwab M, editor. Encyclopedia of Cancer. Springer Berlin Heidelberg; 2009. pp. 2342–3.

[76] Li C-C, Woo S-B. Understanding the pathobiology of head and neck squamous cell carcinoma. Current Oral Health Reports. 2014;1(3):196–203.

[77] van Kempen PMW, van Bockel L, Braunius WW, Moelans CB, van Olst M, de Jong R, et al. HPV-positive oropharyngeal squamous cell carcinoma is associated with TIMP3 and CADM1 promoter hypermethylation. Cancer Medicine. 2014;3(5):1185–96.

[78] Pelosof L, Yerram SR, Ahuja N, Delmas A, Danilova L, Herman JG, et al. CHFR silencing or microsatellite instability is associated with increased antitumor activity of docetaxel or gemcitabine in colorectal cancer. International Journal of Cancer. 2014;134(3):596–605.

[79] Han YH, Hamid MRA, Telisinghe PU, Hussin JBH, Mabruk M. Overexpression of EGFR protein in Bruneian lung cancer patients. Asian Pacific Journal of Cancer Prevention. 2015;16(1):233.

[80] Tepper SR, Zuo Z, Khattri A, Heitmann J, Heß J, Seiwert T. Abstract 1847: Influence of growth factors on resistance to EGFR inhibitor treatment in HNSCC—Temsirolimus as a potential concept. Cancer Research. 2014;74(19 Supplement):1847.

[81] Aigner A, Butscheid M, Kunkel P, Krause E, Lamszus K, Wellstein A, et al. An FGF-binding protein (FGF-BP) exerts its biological function by parallel paracrine stimulation of tumor cell and endothelial cell proliferation through FGF-2 release. International Journal of Cancer. 2001;15;92(4):510–7.

[82] Rettig WJ, Garin-Chesa P, Healey JH, Su SL, Ozer HL, Schwab M, et al. Regulation and heteromeric structure of the fibroblast activation protein in normal and transformed cells of mesenchymal and neuroectodermal origin. Cancer Research. 1993 Jul 15;53(14):3327–35.

[83] Kashyap MK, Marimuthu A, Kishore CJH, Peri S, Keerthikumar S, Prasad TSK, et al. Genomewide mRNA profiling of esophageal squamous cell carcinoma for identification of cancer biomarkers. Cancer Biology and Therapy. 2009;8(1):36–46.

[84] Ayoub C, Wasylyk C, Li Y, Thomas E, Marisa L, Robe A, et al. ANO1 amplification and expression in HNSCC with a high propensity for future distant metastasis and its functions in HNSCC cell lines. British Journal of Cancer. 2010;103(5):715–26.

[85] Huang F, Wong X, Jan LY. International union of basic and clinical pharmacology. LXXXV: calcium-activated chloride channels. *Pharmacological Reviews*. 2012;64(1):1–15.

[86] Almeida LO, Abrahao AC, Rosselli-Murai LK, Giudice FS, Zagni C, Leopoldino AM, et al. NFkappaB mediates cisplatin resistance through histone modifications in head and neck squamous cell carcinoma (HNSCC). FEBS Open Bio. 2014;4:96–104.

[87] Tao Y-F, Xu L-X, Lu J, Cao L, Li Z-H, Hu S-Y, et al. Metallothionein III (MT3) is a putative tumor suppressor gene that is frequently inactivated in pediatric acute myeloid leukemia by promoter hypermethylation. Journal of Translational Medicine. 2014;12(1):182.

[88] Panda S, Beena V, Sivakumar R, Choudhary K, Nalinakumari K, Sathyan S, et al. Microsatellite instability in D2S123 flanking the hMSH2 gene in oral squamous cell carcinoma in South India. Clinical Cancer Investigation Journal. 2015;4(1):22.

[89] de Souza MVR, Servato JPS, Loyola AM, Cardoso SV, Chammas R, Liu F-T, et al. Expression of APC protein during tongue malignant transformation in galectin-3-deficient mice challenged by the carcinogen 4-nitroqunililne-n-oxide. International Journal of Clinical and Experimental Pathology. 2014;7(6):3255–63.

[90] Castilho RM, Gutkind JS. The Wnt/β-catenin signaling circuitry in head and neck cancer. In: Burtness B, Golemis EA, editors. Molecular Determinants of Head and Neck Cancer. Current Cancer Research. New York: Springer; 2014. pp. 199–214.

[91] Paluszczak J, Sarbak J, Kostrzewska-Poczekaj M, Kiwerska K, Jarmuż-Szymczak M, Grenman R, et al. The negative regulators of Wnt pathway—DACH1, DKK1, and WIF1 are methylated in oral and oropharyngeal cancer and WIF1 methylation predicts shorter survival. Tumour Biology. 2014 2014/12/07:1–7.

[92] Komiya Y, Habas R. Wnt signal transduction pathways. Organogenesis. 2008;4(2):68–75.

[93] Supic G, Kozomara R, Jovic N, Zeljic K, Magic Z. Hypermethylation of RUNX3 but not WIF1 gene and its association with stage and nodal status of tongue cancers. Oral Diseases. 2011 Nov;17(8):794–800.

[94] Carvalho AL, Chuang A, Jiang W-W, Lee J, Begum S, Poeta L, et al. Deleted in colorectal cancer is a putative conditional tumor-suppressor gene inactivated by promoter

hypermethylation in head and neck squamous cell carcinoma. Cancer Research. 2006 Oct 1, 2006;66(19):9401–7.

[95] Kaur J, Demokan S, Tripathi SC, Macha MA, Begum S, Califano JA, et al. Promoter hypermethylation in Indian primary oral squamous cell carcinoma. International Journal of Cancer. 2010;127(10):2367–73.

[96] Xiao C, Wang L, Zhu L, Zhang C, Zhou J. Secreted frizzled-related protein 2 is epigenetically silenced and functions as a tumor suppressor in oral squamous cell carcinoma. Molecular Medicine Reports. 2014;10(5):2293–8.

[97] Demokan S, Chang X, Chuang A, Mydlarz WK, Kaur J, Huang P, et al. KIF1A and EDNRB are differentially methylated in primary HNSCC and salivary rinses. International Journal of Cancer. 2010;127(10):2351–9.

[98] Okada Y, Yamazaki H, Sekine-Aizawa Y, Hirokawa N. The neuron-specific kinesin superfamily protein KIF1A is a unique monomeric motor for anterograde axonal transport of synaptic vesicle precursors. Cell. 1995;81(5):769–80.

[99] Smollich M, Wulfing P. Targeting the endothelin system: novel therapeutic options in gynecological, urological and breast cancers. Expert Review of Anticancer Therapy. 2008 Sept;8(9):1481–93.

[100] Yan C, Kim YW, Ha YS, Kim IY, Kim YJ, Yun SJ, et al. RUNX3 methylation as a predictor for disease progression in patients with non-muscle-invasive bladder cancer. Journal of Surgical Oncology. 2012 Mar 15;105(4):425–30.

[101] Kim W-J, Kim E-J, Jeong P, Quan C, Kim J, Li Q-L, et al. RUNX3 inactivation by point mutations and aberrant DNA methylation in bladder tumors. Cancer Research. 2005;65(20):9347–54.

[102] Shigematsu H, Suzuki M, Takahashi T, Miyajima K, Toyooka S, Shivapurkar N, et al. Aberrant methylation of HIN-1 (high in normal-1) is a frequent event in many human malignancies. International Journal of Cancer. 2005 Feb 10;113(4):600–4.

[103] Yu Y, Yin D, Hoque MO, Cao B, Jia Y, Yang Y, et al. AKT signaling pathway activated by HIN-1 methylation in non-small cell lung cancer. Tumour Biology. 2012 Apr; 33(2):307–14.

[104] Krop I, Player A, Tablante A, Taylor-Parker M, Lahti-Domenici J, Fukuoka J, et al. Frequent HIN-1 promoter methylation and lack of expression in multiple human tumor types. Molecular Cancer Res. 2004 Sep;2(9):489–94.

[105] Mancuso M, Matassa DS, Conte M, Colella G, Rana G, Fucci L, et al. H3K4 histone methylation in oral squamous cell carcinoma. Acta Biochimica Polonica. 2009;56(3): 405–10.

[106] Gannon OM, Merida de Long L, Endo-Munoz L, Hazar-Rethinam M, Saunders NA. Dysregulation of the repressive H3K27 trimethylation mark in head and neck squa-

mous cell carcinoma contributes to dysregulated squamous differentiation. Clinical Cancer Research.2013;19(2):428–41.

[107] Dicker AJ, Serewko MM, Dahler AL, Khanna KK, Kaur P, Li A, et al. Functional characterization of cultured cells derived from an intraepidermal carcinoma of the skin (IEC-1). Experimental Cell Research. 2000 Aug 1;258(2):352–60.

[108] Almeida LO, Abrahao AC, Rosselli-Murai LK, Giudice FS, Zagni C, Leopoldino AM, et al. NFκB mediates cisplatin resistance through histone modifications in head and neck squamous cell carcinoma (HNSCC). FEBS Open Bio. 2014;4(0):96–104.

[109] Huang B, Yang X-D, Lamb A, Chen L-F. Posttranslational modifications of NF-kappaB: another layer of regulation for NF-kappaB signaling pathway. Cell Signalling. 2010;22(9):1282–90.

[110] Nakayama K. Growth and progression of melanoma and non-melanoma skin cancers regulated by ubiquitination. Pigment Cell and Melanoma Research. 2010;23(3):338–51.

[111] Hamamoto R, Saloura V, Nakamura Y. Critical roles of non-histone protein lysine methylation in human tumorigenesis. Nature Reviews. Cancer. 2015;15(2):110–24.

[112] Nohata N, Hanazawa T, Kinoshita T, Okamoto Y, Seki N. MicroRNAs function as tumor suppressors or oncogenes: aberrant expression of microRNAs in head and neck squamous cell carcinoma. Auris, Nasus, Larynx. 2013 Apr;40(2):143–9.

[113] Yan B, Broek R, Saleh A, Mehta A, Waes C. Signaling networks of activated oncogenic and altered tumor suppressor genes in head and neck cancer. Journal of Carcinogenesis and Mutagenesis. 2013;7:21–3.

[114] Severino P, Bruggemann H, Andreghetto FM, Camps C, KlingbeilMde F, de Pereira WO, et al. MicroRNA expression profile in head and neck cancer: HOX-cluster embedded microRNA-196a and microRNA-10b dysregulation implicated in cell proliferation. BMC Cancer. 2013;13:533.

[115] Tu HF, Lin SC, Chang KW. MicroRNA aberrances in head and neck cancer: pathogenetic and clinical significance. Current Opinion in Otolaryngology and Head and Neck Surgery. 2013 Apr;21(2):104–11.

[116] Kumar B, Yadav A, Lang J, Teknos TN, Kumar P. Dysregulation of microRNA-34a expression in head and neck squamous cell carcinoma promotes tumor growth and tumor angiogenesis. PloS One. 2012;7(5):e37601.

[117] Datta J, Smith A, Lang JC, Islam M, Dutt D, Teknos TN, et al. microRNA-107 functions as a candidate tumor-suppressor gene in head and neck squamous cell carcinoma by downregulation of protein kinase Cvarepsilon. Oncogene. 2012 Sept 6;31(36): 4045–53.

[118] Lee Y, Yang X, Huang Y, Fan H, Zhang Q, Wu Y, et al. Network modeling identifies molecular functions targeted by mir-204 to suppress head and neck tumor metastasis. PLoS Computational Biology. 2010;6(4):e1000730.

[119] Malek E, Jagannathan S, Driscoll JJ. Correlation of long non-coding RNA expression with metastasis, drug resistance and clinical outcome in cancer. Oncotarget. 2014;5(18):8027–38.

[120] Yao Y, Li J, Wang L. Large intervening non-coding RNA HOTAIR is an indicator of poor prognosis and a therapeutic target in human cancers. International Journal of Molecular Sciences. 2014;15(10):18985–99.

[121] Frith M, Bailey T, Kasukawa T, Mignone F, Kummerfeld S, Madera M, et al. Discrimination of non-protein-coding transcripts from protein-coding mRNA. RNA Biol. 2006;3:40–8.

[122] Tsai M-C, Manor O, Wan Y, Mosammaparast N, Wang JK, Lan F, et al. Long noncoding RNA as modular scaffold of histone modification complexes. Science. 2010;329(5992):689–93.

[123] Marques Howarth M, Simpson D, Ngok SP, Nieves B, Chen R, Siprashvili Z, et al. Long noncoding RNA EWSAT1-mediated gene repression facilitates Ewing sarcoma oncogenesis. Journal of Clinical Investigation. 2014;124(12):5275–90.

[124] Smolle M, Uranitsch S, Gerger A, Pichler M, Haybaeck J. Current status of long non-coding RNAs in human cancer with specific focus on colorectal cancer. International Journal of Molecular Sciences. 2014;15(8):13993–4013.

[125] Amaral PP, Clark MB, Gascoigne DK, Dinger ME, Mattick JS. lncRNAdb: a reference database for long noncoding RNAs. Nucleic Acids Research. 2011;39(Database issue):D146-D51.

[126] Massone S, Ciarlo E, Vella S, Nizzari M, Florio T, Russo C, et al. NDM29, a RNA polymerase III-dependent non coding RNA, promotes amyloidogenic processing of APP and amyloid beta secretion. Biochimica et Biophysica Acta. 2012 Jul;1823(7):1170–7.

[127] Sánchez Y, Huarte M. Long non-coding RNAs: challenges for diagnosis and therapies. Nucleic Acid Therapeutics. 2013;23(1):15–20.

[128] Lakhotia SC. Long non-coding RNAs coordinate cellular responses to stress. Wiley Interdisciplinary Reviews RNA. 2012 Nov–Dec;3(6):779–96.

[129] Verma M. Epigenome-Wide Association Studies (EWAS) in cancer. Current Genomics. 2012;13(4):308–13.

[130] Brait M, Sidransky D. Cancer epigenetics: above and beyond. Toxicology Mechanisms and Methods. 2011;21(4):275–88. PubMed PMID: PMC3309610.

[131] Hoke HA. Enhancers and super-enhancers in human disease and therapy. Massachusetts Institute of Technology; 2014.

[132] Ho AS, Turcan S, Chan TA. Epigenetic therapy: use of agents targeting deacetylation and methylation in cancer management. Onco Targets and Therapy. 2013 03/21;6:223–32.

[133] Li C, Zang Y, Sen M, Leeman-Neill RJ, Grandis JR, Johnson DE. Bortezomib up-regulates activated signal transducer and activator of transcription-3 and synergizes with inhibitors of signal transducer and activator of transcription-3 to promote head and neck squamous cell carcinoma cell death. Molecular Cancer Therapeutics. 2009 07/28;8(8):2211–20.

[134] Nelson NJ. Genetic Events in head and neck squamous cell carcinoma revealed. Journal of the National Cancer Institute. 2013 Dec 4, 2013;105(23):1766–8.

[135] Martins MD, Castilho RM. Histones: controlling tumor signaling circuitry. Journal of Carcinogenesis and Mutagenesis. 2013;1(Suppl 5):1.

[136] Dawson Mark A, Kouzarides T. Cancer epigenetics: from mechanism to therapy. Cell. 2012 7/6/;150(1):12–27.

Chapter 4

The Role of Cancer Stem Cells in Head and Neck Squamous Cell Carcinoma and Its Clinical Implications

Kaveh Karimnejad, Nathan Lindquist and Reigh-Yi Lin

Additional information is available at the end of the chapter

http://dx.doi.org/10.5772/61151

Abstract

Worldwide, more than 550, 000 new cases of head and neck squamous cell carcinoma (HNSCC) are estimated to occur annually, making it the sixth most common human malignancy. Since their discovery in 2007, cancer stem cells (CSCs) in HNSCC have garnered increased interest secondary to their properties of tumorigenicity, differenti- ation, proliferation, and self-renewal. CSCs are intrinsically more resistant to tradi- tional treatments such as radiation and chemotherapy, contributing to potential metastasis and recurrence of HNSCC. This chapter focuses first on normal head and neck stem cells, providing background for the discussion of a number of topics pertaining to the study of HNSCC CSCs including molecular biomarkers and clinical implications. Continued research to elucidate the properties of CSCs will undoubt- edly expand our knowledge surrounding the pathogenesis, metastasis, and relapse of HNSCC. Ultimately, a better understanding of CSC biomarkers, signaling pathways, and mechanisms of resistance will improve therapies and patient outcomes through targeted interventions.

Keywords: Head and neck squamous cell carcinoma, Stem cells, Cancer stem cells, Chemoresistance, Metastasis

1. Introduction

In the United States, over 53, 000 new cases of head and neck squamous cell carcinoma (HNSCC) are estimated to occur each year, with roughly 11, 000 deaths annually [1]. Across the globe, HNSCC has an annual incidence of over 550, 000 cases, making it the sixth most common cancer worldwide. HNSCC accounts for 90% of the malignancies in the head and neck region, affecting the nasal vestibule, nasal cavity, paranasal sinuses, nasopharynx, lips, oral cavity, oropharynx, pharynx, hypopharynx, and larynx. The foundation of treatment for head and neck cancer has been surgery and radiation therapy, while chemotherapy may also be employed as an adjunctive treatment. Advancements in surgical technique, radiation strategies and technologies, as well as chemotherapeutic drugs have led to improvements in patient's overall quality of life. However, the prognosis for HNSCC has improved only marginally over the past thirty years, with the five-year survival rate remaining at 50% [2-4]. Even after standard therapy, patients with HNSCC exhibit relatively high rates of local recurrence, regional cervical lymph node recurrence, and to a lesser degree distant metastasis, all of which contribute to significant morbidity and mortality [5]. Often, these recurrences and metastases are more resistant to traditional treatment modalities such as chemoradiation. Unfortunately, primary site recurrence occurs in 10-30% of all patients [6].

Traditional approaches to understanding and treating HNSCC are based on the stochastic model of cancer, where all tumor cells are identical (Figure 1). More recently, the cancer stem cell (CSC) hypothesis has gained increasing traction in explaining tumorigenesis [7]. This theory proposes that cancer maintains a hierarchical order of cells, with only a small subpopulation of CSCs capable of tumor initiation, propagation, and regeneration [8]. Conventional therapies that target rapidly cycling cells are less effective in killing CSCs. CSCs also display increased intrinsic resistance to chemotherapy and radiation therapy. As a result, CSCs are likely to contribute to cancer relapse.

This review aims to provide a succinct yet thorough overview of our current basis for the CSC hypothesis as it pertains to HNSCC. We will start with a brief discussion of the normal epithelium of the head and neck region as well as our current understanding of normal endogenous stem cells of the head and neck region. Evidence for the CSC hypothesis of

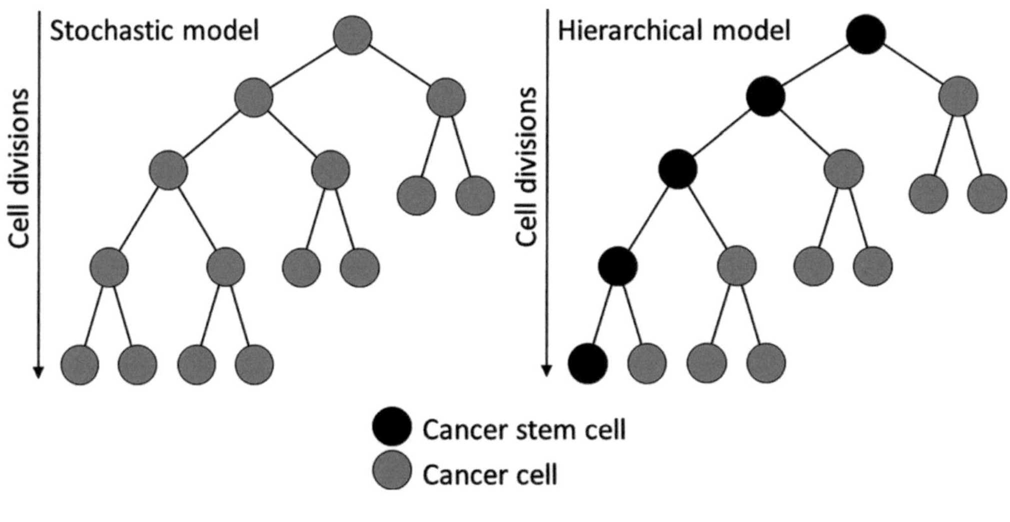

Figure 1. In the stochastic model, all tumor cells have equal abilities to propagate, initiate tumors, and seed metastases. The heterogeneity of tumors in this model is derived from spontaneous phenotypic shifts. The emerging cancer stem cell hypothesis dictates the hierarchical model, in which asymmetric division results in specific and well-defined populations of cancer stem cells and other cancer cells that do not initiate tumors or seed metastases. These cells may consist of populations with decreased proliferative ability (i.e., transit-amplifying cells) or post-mitotic differentiated cells with no further proliferative ability or activity.

HNSCC will include a discussion of the prospective markers for CSCs in HNSCC, as well as a closer look at the cellular regulation of these CSCs and the clinical implications of these cancer- initiating and propagating cells.

2. Head and neck stem cells in normal tissues

Stem cells are unique in their ability to maintain self-renewal, differentiate into multiple lineage types in the same tissue, and display a high degree of proliferative potential [9]. The somatic stem cell microenvironment or cellular "niche" is vital in maintaining the delicate distinction between self-renewal and uncontrolled proliferation of stem cells [10]. Stem cells and the extracellular matrix secrete factors to maintain the microenvironment, while inhibitory signals from this local microenvironment provide necessary control of proliferation and differentiation to sustain this important subpopulation of cells [11, 12]. Importantly, these quiescent, undifferentiated somatic stem cells also depend on the niche for the transient stimulatory signals necessary for cell division and tissue regeneration [13]. Unlike most of the gastrointestinal tract, which contains a simple epithelial layer to allow for increased absorption, the oral cavity, pharynx, and esophagus are covered by a stratified epithelium that is more similar in structure to other tissues such as skin [14]. The stratified epithelium is composed of multiple layers of cell types oriented in order of increasing differentiation from basal to superficial.

In the normal squamous stratified epithelium, stem cells are located in the basal layer. To replenish the more superficial layers, these stem cells divide asymmetrically to self-renew and produce cells to undergo subsequent differentiation and amplification [11]. Cell division in stratified squamous epithelium results in differentiation, superficial cellular movement, stratification, and ultimately, tissue turnover. In the stratified squamous epithelium, for example, a layer of small, cuboidal, basal stem cells are responsible for cell division and regeneration [15]. Moving superficially, these committed cells further differentiate to increase keratin filament production, flatten, and decrease the size and volume of the nucleus and organelles. The most superficial (corneal or superficial) layers of the oral mucosa demonstrate cell flattening, mem- brane thickening, decreased desmosomes, and eventual sloughing of cells into the oral cavity [16]. The hierarchical normal oral epithelium is renewed approximately every 14–24 days [17]. Increasingly, endogenous oral cavity stem cells are theorized to precede CSCs, as these are the only cells with life span sufficient to accumulate the genetic mutations necessary for malignant transformation [18].

3. Head and neck stem cell markers

In contrast to other tissues or organ systems, relatively few markers have been identified or characterized for normal endogenous stem cells of the head and neck region. To date, most of our knowledge of normal head and neck stem cells is based largely on work on oral epithelial stem cells (OESCs) and corollaries from the skin and hair follicle, which also maintain a squamous stratified epithelium.

In the 1960s, the first experiments to identify potential stem cells in the oral mucosa utilized pulse-chase experiments with tritiated-thymidine ($_3$H-TdR) to elucidate cell turnover rates in the skin and oral mucosa and identify label-retaining cells in the basal layer [19]. Of the few candidate cell surface markers for OESCs, most are also expressed in other normal oral epithelial basal cells, meaning that much of the research involving OESC markers has involved purification rather than isolation of these cells [20]. Such work is often accomplished based on sorting for cell markers and performing subsequent *in vitro* experiments to test the self-renewal and proliferative properties of these subpopulations. So far, notable candidate oral stem cell markers include keratins K5, 14, 15, and 19, β1- and α6-integrins, integrin $\alpha_6\beta_4$, melanoma chondroitin sulfate proteoglycan (MCSP), p75$_{NGFR}$, B-cell-specific Moloney murine leukemia virus integration site 1 (BMI1), and the p63 transcription factor (Table 1) [20-37].

Aida *et al.* performed telomere analysis of different cell types in normal lingual epithelium to calculate normalized telomere:centromere ratios (NTCRs). Overall, the basal cell group demonstrated the largest NTCR, with a smaller subgroup of these cells maintaining an exceptionally large NTCR, suggesting the presence of stem cells. In general, stem cells are thought to maintain relatively longer telomeres due to a lower telomere turnover rate as well as the potential for telomere upregulation. In addition, samples from older patients contained relatively shorter telomeres, confirming a measurable age-related progression. Finally, immunohistochemistry confirmed the presence of p27, p63, and K19 in the basal layer with relatively scant staining for Ki-67, a well-known marker of cell proliferation [22].

In one study, the magnetic separation of oral human keratinocytes yielded a fraction of α6β +CD71 cells that could regenerate a stratified oral epithelial equivalent *in vitro*. Unlike either of the α6β +CD71+ or or $\alpha_6\beta$ keratinocyte groups, $\alpha_6\beta_+CD71_-$ cells also expressed the candidate stem cell markers p63 and Keratin 19 and were negative for two recognized markers of differentiation: cytokeratin 10 or involucrin [23].

Tao *et al.* demonstrate a method of enriching a subpopulation containing both potential stem cells and transit amplifying cells through integrin-β1 adherence to collagen IV. While their subsequent study of p63 expression could not confirm specificity for stem cells in the basal layer, the ΔNp63α and ΔNp63β isoforms may be more specific markers for undifferentiated or immature cells [21].

Through cell lineage mapping, Hogan and coworkers noted a $K14_+K5_+Trp63_+Sox2_+$ subpopulation of long-term stem or progenitor cells located outside the taste buds that are capable of differentiating into both mature taste bud receptor cells as well as keratinocytes. The authors suggest that a similar model may apply to the taste buds of the circumvallate papillae and soft palate, and that their work may prove a model system for future study of these endogenous stem cells [24]. This same group isolated a population of undifferentiated tongue basal cells using Krt5-eGFP transgenic mice that demonstrated self-renewal and differentiation to stratified keratinized epithelial cells *in vitro*.

http://dx.doi.org/10.5772/61151

Candidate Normal Stem Cell Marker	Site(s) Studied	Function and Significance in Stem Cell Biology	References
Keratin 5	Mouse tongue and soft palate	ntermediate filament protein expressed by basal epithelial cells, only small fraction may actually replicate	[24,29,31]
Keratin 14	Mouse tongue and oral mucosa	Intermediate filament protein expressed by basal epithelial cells, only small fraction of these cells may actually replicate	[24,29,32]
Keratin 15	Human hard palate	Intermediate filament protein, marker of stem cells in hair follicle bulge, expressed in deep tips of palatal epithelial papillae	[33]
Keratin 19	Human hard palate and gingiva	Intermediate filament protein, stem cell marker for cells of hair follicle	[22,23,34,35]
β1-integrin	Cultured human epidermal, buccal, and gingival cells	Important in adhesion to extracellular matrix proteins, increased in cells with higher colony-forming efficiency	[21,36]
α6β4-integrin	Human hard palate and gingiva	Important in adhesion to basement membrane, expressed on α6β4 CD71 basal cells capable of oral epithelium regeneration	[23,33,34]
MCSP	Human hard palate	Cellular surface proteoglycan associated with migration and invasion of melanoma cells, important for maintenance of patterned distribution and clustering of epidermal stem cells	[20,33,37]
p75NGFR	Human esophageal, buccal, gingival, and laryngeal epithelium	Low-affinity neurotrophin receptor in TNF receptor superfamily important in proliferation, cell migration, and tissue regeneration	[25-28]
p63	Rat palate and oral mucosa, human tongue, gingival and buccal epithelium	Transcription factor with multiple isoforms responsible for epidermal stem cell maintenance and regulation	[21,22,24,34]
BMI1	Mouse lingual epithelium	Protein involved with epithelial cell maintenance, proliferation, and tissue regeneration	[29]

Table 1. The function and significance of candidate normal stem cell markers in the head and neck region.

The low-affinity neurotrophin receptor $p75_{NGFR}$ is a member of the tumor necrosis factor receptor superfamily and has effects in cell survival, apoptosis, and intercellular signaling [25]. It has been put forth as a possible stem cell marker for neural crest, mesenchymal, esophageal, oral mucosa [25], and most recently laryngeal epithelium [25, 26]. In addition, $p75_{NGFR}$-positive basal keratinocytes are able to migrate and initiate regeneration of damaged buccal epithelium [27]. Furthermore, expression of $p75_{NGFR}$ has been shown to be closely related to CSCs in esophageal squamous cell carcinoma as well as laryngeal squamous cell carcinoma [26, 28].

Recent interest in lingual epithelial stem cells has provided some evidence that keratins K5 and K14 may not be specific stem cell markers in this system. Ueno and coworkers utilized immunostaining to reveal that only a small fraction of these keratins K14/K5-positive cells were actually replicating to supply epithelial cells [29]. Rather, this group identified a group of BMI1-positive stem cells that maintain the epithelial cells and can regenerate after irradia- tion-induced tissue injury. Curiously, these potential stem cells were located in the second or third epithelial layer of the interpapillary pit of the filiform papillae. Increasingly, BMI1 is viewed as a candidate marker for CSCs of the head and neck, with the potential for prognostic value based on the location of this intracellular oncoprotein [30].

MCSP, melanoma-associated chondroitin sulfate proteoglycan; NGFR, nerve growth factor receptor; TNF, tumor necrosis factor; BMI1, B-cell-specific Moloney murine leukemia virus integration site 1

4. Origin of head and neck cancer stem cells

In most instances, HNSCC is caused by the accumulation of multiple genetic mutations based on genetic predisposition, which is induced by environmental factors such as tobacco and alcohol abuse or persistent human papilloma virus infection [38]. However, the alterations of multiple molecular and cellular pathways that lead to the development and recurrence of HNSCC are still not well understood. Recently, recurrence and therapeutic resistance of HNSCC has been attributed to a subpopulation of self-sustaining, tumor-initiating CSCs. CSCs are defined by several exclusive features that allow propagation as well as tumor formation and maintenance. These features are: (1) differentiation, giving rise to heterogeneous progeny; (2) self-renewal, which maintains a pool of stem cells which can expand; and (3) homeostatic control, which accounts for tissue specificity [4].

Multiple possible origins for CSCs have been proposed wherein a population of self-renewing cells are formed, leading to tumorigenesis (Figure 2) [39]. In one such scenario, normal stem cells undergo mutations that diminish restraint on replication, thereby creating CSCs that are unresponsive to environmental or intrinsic controls on self-renewal. Another potential source of CSCs are the more differentiated progenitor cells, also known as transit-amplifying cells, which maintain a more limited role in self-renewal yet are far more numerous than stem cells. A third motif of CSC generation explains that well-differentiated, mature cells undergo mutations to dedifferentiate and obtain greater self-renewal potential [5]. There is evidence that these dedifferentiated HNSCC cells may undergo epithelial-mesenchymal transition and invasion, leading to the development of cells with CSC- or mesenchymal characteristics [40].

5. Initial clues to the concept of head and neck cancer stem cells

The first "leukemia-initiating" CSCs were identified in 1994 by Dick and co-workers through their work with acute myeloid leukemia [41]. In 2003, Al-Hajj *et al.* reported the first CSCs in a solid tumor by separating a tumorigenic subpopulation of breast cancer cells based on the surface cell markers $CD44_{+}/CD24_{-/low}$ [42]. In 2007, a landmark study by Prince *et al.* described a subpopulation of $CD44_{+}$ tumor-initiating cells isolated from HNSCC, although the cell surface markers CD44s and CD44v6 were subsequently described in a majority of normal head and neck tissues as well as HNSCC [43, 44]. Other subpopulations of tumor-initiating cells have since been identified in HNSCC that also fulfill the criteria for CSCs. Furthermore, several of the putative markers of these CSC subpopulations have been linked to cancer recurrence and therapeutic resistance, augmenting the evidence for the CSC hypothesis in HNSCC. Recent interest in the identification of new and improved biomarkers for HNSCC CSCs has spiked due to the prospect of using these tools to improve treatment approaches and overall mortality in this deadly disease.

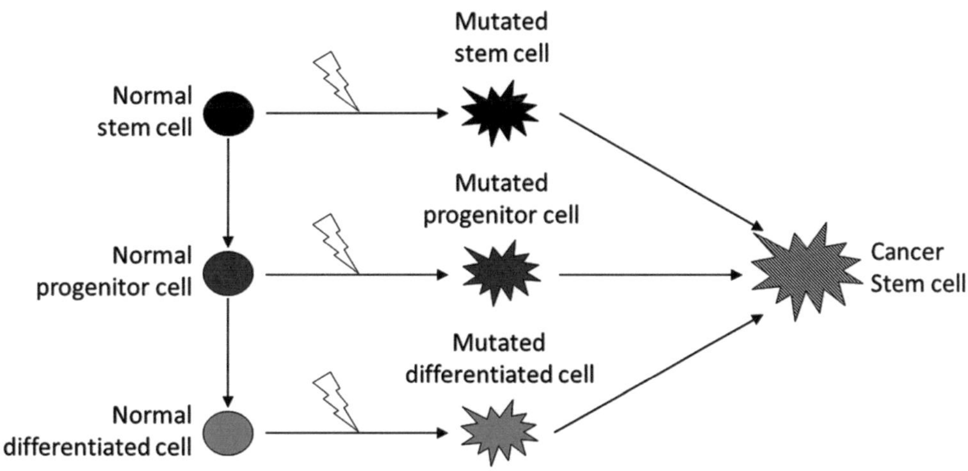

Figure 2. Potential origins for cancer stem cells include normal stem cells, progenitor cells, or fully differentiated cells. To give rise to cancer stem cells, the progenitor and fully differentiated cells acquire mutations to reactivate genes responsible for increased proliferative activity, cell-division, and dedifferentiation.

6. Cancer stem cell assays

The isolation and identification of CSCs is a hefty experimental challenge, as there is no established protocol to verify putative CSCs. Current experimental goals aim to satisfy the CSC criteria of both self-renewal as well as the capacity to develop heterogeneous cell lineages capable of forming tumors identical to the original [45]. Isolation strategies attempt to exploit the unique properties of CSCs that distinguish them from their differentiated progeny. Such capacities include the efflux of vital dyes by multidrug transporters, enzymatic activity, sphere-forming capacity in low attachment conditions, and the expression of cell surface antigens [46]. There are currently four main strategies for isolation of CSCs: (1) detection of side-population phenotypes by Hoechst 33342 exclusion, (2) sphere-formation assays, (3) assessment of aldehyde dehydrogenase (ALDH) activity, and (4) identification of CSC-specific cell surface markers [45]. To date, the most common modality in identifying HNSCC CSCs relies upon the expression of membrane cell surface antigens present in stem-like cells. As a result, most potential CSC populations are detected by immunohistochemistry or flow cytometry. Many of these antigens were originally put forth as potential targets as a result of their expression in normal stem cells [47, 48]. Herein, we present a review of the most promising putative HNSCC CSC markers: CD44, CD133, and ALDH. We also include a discussion of CD24 and CD10.

Putative Cancer Stem Cell Markers in HNSCC Sites Studied	**Biological Function**	**Significance in HNSCC Stem Cell Biology**	**References**
CD44	Surface glycoprotein involved in cell migration and adhesion	Showed the ability to regenerate tumor *in vivo* but also abundantly expressed in normal squamous epithelia of the head and neck. Associated with Snail (chemoresistance and radioresistance) as well as high coexpression of BMI1 (important for self-renewal and tumorigenesis)	[43,44,49,50,55]
CD133 (Prominin 1)	Transmembrane glycoprotein localized on membrane protrusions and microvilli	Correlated with lymph node metastases and decreased overall survival	[51,52,54,55]
ALDH	Intracellular enzyme most commonly found in the liver. ALDH detoxifies intracellular aldehydes through oxidation	Tumor cells expressing relatively high levels of ALDH have increased tumorigenicity, stem-cell-related genes, drug-resistant genes, and EMT-related genes. Associated with high co-expression of Snail protein, which is an EMT regulator and key factor in self- renewal and tumorigenicity	[47,56,65]

Putative Cancer Stem Cell Markers in HNSCC Sites Studied	Biological Function	Significance in HNSCC Stem Cell Biology	References
CD24	Mucin adhesion molecule for P-selectin and L1 expressed by pre-B lymphocytes and neutrophils during cell development	Associated with increased proliferation and invasion *in vitro* and tumorigenicity *in vivo*, correlates with increased resistance to chemotherapeutic agents	[47,60,62]
CD10	Zinc-dependent metalloendoprotease that cleaves signaling peptides and is found in a wide range of normal tissues	Described as a potential marker for therapeutic resistance and tumor recurrence in HNSCC	[64]

Table 2. The function, significance, and associations of putative cancer stem cell markers in HNSCC.

7. Putative head and neck cancer stem cell markers

7.1. CD44

CD44 is a surface glycoprotein involved in cell migration and adhesion. Prince *et al.* demonstrated the ability of a subpopulation of $CD44_+$ HNSCC cells to regenerate a tumor *in vivo* after transplantation of as few as $5x10_3$ cells into an immunocompromised mouse model [44]. $CD44_+$ cells have been shown to express a high level of BMI1, a prospective normal stem cell bio- marker that also plays a key role in self-renewal and tumorigenesis in malignancy [49, 50]. While CD44 was the first CSC marker established for HNSCC, its role has since come into question. In contrast to earlier studies involving CD44, recent studies have demonstrated the abundant expression of CD44 in most HNSCC tumor cells. In one such study, CD44 was present in 80-100% of tumor cells [43]. However, according to the *hierarchical model*, only a small subset of cells within malignant tissue that are able to generate tumors should stain positive for CSC markers. Furthermore, high percentages of $CD44_+$ cells have been identified in normal squamous epithelia of the head and neck, with up to 60–95% of normal head and neck epithelial cells demonstrating CD44 positivity. Although the role of CD44 in HNSCC has raised some questions, this protein may still prove a valuable role in the identification of CSCs when used in combination with other markers. In the 2009 study by Chen *et al.*, not only did knockdown of Snail expression in $CD44_+ALDH_+$ cells decrease tumor invasion and colony formation, but it also significantly increased sensitivity to chemotherapy and radiotherapy. Specifically, following seven days of Snail siRNA treatment, the $CD44_+ALDH_+$ CSCs exhibited increased sensitivity to cisplatin and etoposide, and radiotherapy. These findings illustrate the potential utility of CSCs as unique cell targets for both chemotherapy and radiation therapy.

7.2. CD133

First described in 1997, CD133 (Prominin 1) is a transmembrane glycoprotein expressed in several normal stem cell populations and malignancies [51]. CD133 is localized to cellular membrane protrusions and microvilli [52]. It is expressed in several solid malignancies including brain, colon, liver, and lung, and has been purported as a unique, specific marker for sarcomas [38]. In 2007, Zhou *et al.* demonstrated the presence of a $CD133_+$ subpopulation in 3.5% of the native cells from a HEp-2 laryngeal cancer cell line. These $CD133_+$ cells continued to proliferate and expand the tumor cell population in sphere formation assays. In cell culture assays, the majority of terminal cells did not express CD133, a finding consistent with the criteria for CSC self-renewal as well as the capacity to give rise to phenotypically unique tumor daughter cells [53]. More recent studies have supported these findings, suggesting the utility of CD133 as a clinically relevant prognostic marker in HNSCC. Canis *et al.* demonstrated an inversely proportional correlation between CD133 expression in primary tumors and overall survival in addition to a positive correlation between CD133 expression and the presence of lymph node metastases [54]. In addition, Yu *et al.* describe an oral cavity squamous cell carcinoma-derived side population of cells with high expression of CD133 and ALDH showed high tumorigenic capacity [55]. Cell viability assays revealed that these side populations of cells were more chemoresistant to cisplatin, fluorouracil, or doxorubicin treatment when compared to the major population of the same cell line. The researchers hypothesized that CD133 may be crucial to modulation of chemosensitivity. They subsequently performed lentiviral-mediated transduction in the side population of cells, which resulted in significant decrease in expression of CD133 mRNA and protein. The silencing of CD133 decreased the percentage of the side population in the cancer cell lines and decreased *in vivo* tumor growth. Furthermore, cisplatin treatment of the CD133 knockdown population diminished cell invasion and clonogenicity, demonstrating the enhanced sensitivity to chemotherapy by targeting CD133. These findings support the role of HNSCC CSCs as novel therapeutic targets in the development of chemotherapeutic drugs.

7.3. ALDH

ALDH is an intracellular enzyme most commonly found in the liver [47]. ALDH detoxifies intracellular aldehydes through oxidation and may play a role in the differentiation of stem cells by oxidizing retinol into retinoic acid. With regard to cancer, high ALDH activity has been linked to subsets of multiple myeloma and acute myeloid leukemia [56]. Prior to its identification with HNSCC, ALDH was labeled a putative CSC marker in both breast and colon cancer. Ginestier *et al.* successfully used high ALDH activity to identify a tumorigenic breast cancer cell fraction capable of self-renewal and generating heterogeneous tumors. In their study, expression of ALDH as detected by immunohistochemistry correlated with a poorer prognosis for breast carcinomas [57].

Expression of ALDH1 in inflammatory breast cancer has been put forth as an independent predictor of early metastasis and decreased survival [58]. In 2009, Chen *et al.* published the first study demonstrating that cells of $ALDH1_+$ lineage have CSC properties and play a role in self- renewal in HNSCC [3]. In a study by Clay *et al.*, HNSCC cells were categorized and isolated based on either high or low ALDH activity and subsequently implanted into immunocompromised mice. Cells with relatively high levels of ALDH represented a small percentage of cells (1% to 7.8%), but gave rise to tumors from as few as 500 cells in 53% of implantations. In contrast, only 8% of similar implantations with cells expressing low levels of ALDH formed tumor. As a result, ALDH appears to be a relatively selective marker for HNSCC CSCs [56]. In a similar study, 87% of implantations with 1000 $ALDH_+CD44_+$ HNSCC cells generated tumors, compared to only 13% of $ALDH_-CD44_-$ cell implantations, despite utilizing ten times more cells: 10, 000 [59]. $ALDH_+$ cells have also been shown to exhibit higher expression levels of stem cell-related, drug-resistance-associated, and epithelial-mesenchymal-transformation-related (EMT) genes such as Snail [3]. In fact, Snail protein overexpression transformed $ALDH_-$ cells to $ALDH_+$ cells, resulting in increased invasion and tumorigenic properties [65]. Given this association with Snail and EMT, as well as the ability to recapitulate tumors in high percentages after *in vivo* implantation in multiple studies, ALDH may be the most well-established HNSCC CSC marker to date.

7.4. CD24 and CD10

CD24 is a mucin adhesion molecule for P-selectin and L1 expressed by pre-B lymphocytes and neutrophils during cell development [47, 60]. CD24 expression has been shown to increase tumor cell proliferation and further shown to regulate multiple cell properties which contribute to tumor growth and metastasis [60]. It has been correlated with increased spread of breast cancer and has been further identified as a putative CSC marker in pancreatic, ovarian, and colorectal cancers [61, 62]. CD24 has also been associated with tumorigenesis, tumor progression, and malignant transformation of stomach and gallbladder cancers [63]. In a study by Han *et al.* $CD24_+CD44_+$ HNSCC cells were demonstrated to be more proliferative and invasive *in vitro* and more tumorigenic *in vivo.* After implantation in immunodeficient mice, $CD24_+CD44_+$ *cells* formed larger tumors than the $CD24_-CD44_+$ group. $CD24_+CD44_+$ cells were also correlated with slightly increased resistance to chemotherapeutic agents [62]. CD24 is one of the primary surface antigens involved in solid tumors and its role has been established in various human epithelial neoplasias. However, the paucity of research concerning HNSCC precludes its inclu- sion as a CSC biomarker at the present time.

CD10 is a zinc-dependent metalloendoprotease that cleaves signaling peptides and is found in a wide range of normal tissues. It has been described as a potential marker for therapeutic resistance and tumor recurrence in HNSCC [64]. As the field of CSCs remains in its infancy, further investigation regarding the roles of CD24 and CD10 will better elucidate the role of these proteins in HNSCC.

8. Clinical relevance of head and neck cancer stem cells

Today, few studies have evaluated patient HNSCC tumors or tissues and the correlation with clinical data and outcomes. One barrier to the establishment of clinically significant CSC markers in the head and neck region is secondary to the convention of amassing malignancies from various upper aerodigestive sites with distinctly diverse embryological and biological characteristics [47]. As a result, there is little definitive data with regard to clinical implications of CSCs within HNSCC, the primary exception being prognostic value. Furthermore, no single biomarker for CSC cells in HNSCC has proven absolute in distinguishing this vital subpopulation. The continued study of current prospective CSC markers in HNSCC, combined with the investigation of putative CSC biomarkers from other malignancies, will undoubtedly augment our knowledge and improve our understanding of the pathogenesis of HNSCC. In addition, further knowledge regarding the biomarkers and regulation of normal, native stem cells in the head and neck region will serve as a strong foundation for oncological research. Ultimately, CSCs may prove to be useful diagnostic and prognostic markers for HNSCC, guiding therapy and treatment through personalized approaches and interventions.

Author details

Kaveh Karimnejad[#], Nathan Lindquist[#], Reigh-Yi Lin[*]

*Address all correspondence to: rlin7@slu.edu

Department of Otolaryngology – Head and Neck Surgery, Saint Louis University School of Medicine, Saint Louis, Missouri, USA

[#] These authors contribute equally to this work.

References

[1] Siegel R, Naishadham D, Jemal A. Cancer statistics, 2013. *CA*: A cancer journal for clinicians. 2013;63(1):11–30.

[2] Anderson RT, Keysar SB, Bowles DW, Glogowska MJ, Astling DP, Morton JJ, et al. The dual pathway inhibitor rigosertib is effective in direct patient tumor xenografts of head and neck squamous cell carcinomas. *Mol Canc Therapeut*. 2013;12(10):1994–2005.

[3] Chen Z. The cancer stem cell concept in progression of head and neck cancer. *J Oncol*. 2009;2009:8.

[4] Bhaijee F, Pepper DJ, Pitman KT, Bell D. Cancer stem cells in head and neck squamous cell carcinoma: a review of current knowledge and future applications. *Head Neck*. 2012;34(6):894–9.

[5] Shah A, Patel S, Pathak J, Swain N, Kumar S. The evolving concepts of cancer stem cells in head and neck squamous cell carcinoma. *Scientific World J*. 2014;2014:8.

[6] Wolf GT. Surgical margins in the genomic era: The Hayes Martin Lecture, 2012. *Arch Otolaryngol Head Neck Surg*. 2012;138(11):1001–13.

[7] Wicha MS, Liu S, Dontu G. Cancer stem cells: an old idea – a paradigm shift. *Canc Res*. 2006;66(4):1883–90; discussion 95–6.

[8] Reya T, Morrison SJ, Clarke MF, Weissman IL. Stem cells, cancer, and cancer stem cells. *Nature*. 2001;414(6859):105–11.

[9] Jordan CT, Guzman ML, Noble M. Cancer Stem Cells. *N Eng J Med*. 2006;355(12): 1253–61.

[10] Li L, Neaves WB. Normal stem cells and cancer stem cells: the niche matters. *Canc Res*. 2006;66(9):4553–7.

[11] Mannelli G, Gallo O. Cancer stem cells hypothesis and stem cells in head and neck cancers. *Canc Treat Rev*. 2012;38(5):515–39.

[12] Scadden DT. The stem-cell niche as an entity of action. *Nature*. 2006;441(7097):1075–9.

[13] Fuchs E, Tumbar T, Guasch G. Socializing with the neighbors: stem cells and their niche. *Cell*. 2004;116(6):769–78.

[14] Squier CA, Kremer MJ. Biology of oral mucosa and esophagus. *J Natl Canc Instit Mono- graphs*. 2001(29):7–15.

[15] Nguyen LV, Vanner R, Dirks P, Eaves CJ. Cancer stem cells: an evolving concept. *Nature Rev Canc*. 2012;12(2):133–43.

[16] Winning TA, Townsend GC. Oral mucosal embryology and histology. *Clinics Dermatol*. 2000;18(5):499–511.

[17] Richard V, Pillai MR. The stem cell code in oral epithelial tumorigenesis: 'the cancer stem cell shift hypothesis'. *Biochim Biophys Acta*. 2010;1806(2):146–62.

[18] Costea DE, Tsinkalovsky O, Vintermyr OK, Johannessen AC, Mackenzie IC. Cancer stem cells – new and potentially important targets for the therapy of oral squamous cell carcinoma. *Oral Dis*. 2006;12(5):443–54.

[19] Cutright DE, Bauer H. Cell renewal in the oral mucosa and skin of the rat. I. Turnover time. *Oral Surg Oral Med Oral Pathol*. 1967;23(2):249–59.

[20] Jones KB, Klein OD. Oral epithelial stem cells in tissue maintenance and disease: the first steps in a long journey. *Int J Oral Sci*. 2013;5(3):121–9.

[21] Tao Q, Qiao B, Lv B, Zheng C, Chen Z, Huang H. p63 and its isoforms as markers of rat oral mucosa epidermal stem cells in vitro. *Cell Biochem Funct*. 2009;27(8):535–41.

[22] Aida J, Izumiyama-Shimomura N, Nakamura K, Ishikawa N, Poon SS, Kammori M, et al. Basal cells have longest telomeres measured by tissue Q-FISH method in lingual epithe- lium. *Exper Gerontol*. 2008;43(9):833–9.

[23] Calenic B, Ishkitiev N, Yaegaki K, Imai T, Costache M, Tovaru M, et al. Characterization of oral keratinocyte stem cells and prospects of its differentiation to oral epithelial equiv- alents. Romanian journal of morphology and embryology = *Rev Roumaine Morphol Embryolog*. 2010;51(4):641–5.

[24] Okubo T, Clark C, Hogan BL. Cell lineage mapping of taste bud cells and keratinocytes in the mouse tongue and soft palate. *Stem Cells* (Dayton, Ohio). 2009;27(2):442–50.

[25] Nakamura T, Endo K, Kinoshita S. Identification of human oral keratinocyte stem/pro- genitor cells by neurotrophin receptor p75 and the role of neurotrophin/p75 signaling. *Stem Cells* (Dayton, Ohio). 2007;25(3):628–38.

[26] Li X, Shen Y, Di B, Li J, Geng J, Lu X, et al. Biological and clinical significance of p75NTR expression in laryngeal squamous epithelia and laryngocarcinoma. *Acta Oto-laryngol*. 2012;132(3):314–24.

[27] Ishii A, Muramatsu T, Lee JM, Higa K, Shinozaki N, Jung HS, et al. Expression of p75 (NGFR), a proliferative and basal cell Marker, in the buccal mucosa epithelium during re- epithelialization. *Acta Histochem Cytochem*. 2014;47(4):145–53.

[28] Huang SD, Yuan Y, Liu XH, Gong DJ, Bai CG, Wang F, et al. Self-renewal and chemother- apy resistance of p75NTR positive cells in esophageal squamous cell carcinomas. *BMC Canc*. 2009;9:9.

[29] Tanaka T, Komai Y, Tokuyama Y, Yanai H, Ohe S, Okazaki K, et al. Identification of stem cells that maintain and regenerate lingual keratinized epithelial cells. *Natur Cell Biol*. 2013;15(5):511–8.

[30] Allegra E, Trapasso S, Pisani D, Puzzo L. The role of BMI1 as a biomarker of cancer stem cells in head and neck cancer: a review. *Oncology*. 2014;86(4):199–205.

[31] Luo X, Okubo T, Randell S, Hogan BL. Culture of endodermal stem/progenitor cells of the mouse tongue. In vitro cellular & developmental biology. *Animal*. 2009;45(1–2):44–54.

[32] Raimondi AR, Molinolo A, Gutkind JS. Rapamycin prevents early onset of tumorigenesis in an oral-specific K-ras and p53 two-hit carcinogenesis model. *Canc Res*. 2009;69 (10):4159–66.

[33] Mackenzie IC. Stem cells in oral mucosal epithelia. *Oral Biosci Med*. 2005;2(2):95–103.

[34] Calenic B, Ishkitiev N, Yaegaki K, Imai T, Kumazawa Y, Nasu M, et al. Magnetic separa- tion and characterization of keratinocyte stem cells from human gingiva. *J Periodontal Res*. 2010;45(6):703–8.

[35] Michel M, Torok N, Godbout MJ, Lussier M, Gaudreau P, Royal A, et al. Keratin 19 as a biochemical marker of skin stem cells in vivo and in vitro: keratin 19 expressing

cells are differentially localized in function of anatomic sites, and their number varies with donor age and culture stage. *J Cell Sci*. 1996;109 (Pt 5):1017–28.

[36] Jones PH, Watt FM. Separation of human epidermal stem cells from transit amplifying cells on the basis of differences in integrin function and expression. *Cell*. 1993;73 (4):713–24.

[37] Legg J, Jensen UB, Broad S, Leigh I, Watt FM. Role of melanoma chondroitin sulphate proteoglycan in patterning stem cells in human interfollicular epidermis. *Development* (Cambridge, England). 2003;130(24):6049–63.

[38] Albers AE, Chen C, Koberle B, Qian X, Klussmann JP, Wollenberg B, et al. Stem cells in squamous head and neck cancer. *Critic Rev Oncol/Hematol*. 2012;81(3):224–40.

[39] Clarke MF, Fuller M. Stem cells and cancer: two faces of eve. *Cell*. 2006;124(6):1111–5.

[40] Chen C, Wei Y, Hummel M, Hoffmann TK, Gross M, Kaufmann AM, et al. Evidence for epithelial-mesenchymal transition in cancer stem cells of head and neck squamous cell carcinoma. *PLoS One*. 2011;6(1):e16466.

[41] Lapidot T, Sirard C, Vormoor J, Murdoch B, Hoang T, Caceres-Cortes J, et al. A cell initiating human acute myeloid leukaemia after transplantation into SCID mice. *Nature*. 1994;367(6464):645–8.

[42] Al-Hajj M, Wicha MS, Benito-Hernandez A, Morrison SJ, Clarke MF. Prospective identi- fication of tumorigenic breast cancer cells. *Proc Natl Acad Sci*. 2003;100(7): 3983–8.

[43] Mack B, Gires O. CD44s and CD44v6 expression in head and neck epithelia. *PLoS One*. 2008;3(10):e3360.

[44] Prince ME, Sivanandan R, Kaczorowski A, Wolf GT, Kaplan MJ, Dalerba P, et al. Identi- fication of a subpopulation of cells with cancer stem cell properties in head and neck squamous cell carcinoma. *Proc Natl Acad Sci*. 2007;104(3):973–8.

[45] Tirino V, Desiderio V, Paino F, De Rosa A, Papaccio F, La Noce M, et al. Cancer stem cells in solid tumors: an overview and new approaches for their isolation and characterization. *FASEB J* : official publication of the Federation of American Societies for Experimental Biology. 2013;27(1):13–24.

[46] Krishnamurthy S, Nör JE. Head and neck cancer stem cells. *J Dental Res*. 2012;91 (4): 334–40.

[47] Allegra E, Trapasso S. Cancer stem cells in head and neck cancer. *OncoTargets Ther*. 2012;5:375–83.

[48] Monroe MM, Anderson EC, Clayburgh DR, Wong MH. Cancer stem cells in head and neck squamous cell carcinoma. *J Oncol*. 2011;2011:762780.

[49] Lessard J, Sauvageau G. Bmi-1 determines the proliferative capacity of normal and leukaemic stem cells. *Nature*. 2003;423(6937):255–60.

[50] Park IK, Morrison SJ, Clarke MF. Bmi1, stem cells, and senescence regulation. *J Clin Invest*. 2004;113(2):175–9.

[51] Yin AH, Miraglia S, Zanjani ED, Almeida-Porada G, Ogawa M, Leary AG, et al. AC133, a novel marker for human hematopoietic stem and progenitor cells. *Blood*. 1997;90 (12):5002–12.

[52] Corbeil D, Marzesco AM, Wilsch-Brauninger M, Huttner WB. The intriguing links between prominin-1 (CD133), cholesterol-based membrane microdomains, remodeling of apical plasma membrane protrusions, extracellular membrane particles, and (neuro) epithelial cell differentiation. *FEBS Lett*. 2010;584(9):1659–64.

[53] Zhou L, Wei X, Cheng L, Tian J, Jiang JJ. CD133, one of the markers of cancer stem cells in Hep-2 cell line. *Laryngoscope*. 2007;117(3):455–60.

[54] Canis M, Lechner A, Mack B, Zengel P, Laubender RP, Koehler U, et al. CD133 is a predictor of poor survival in head and neck squamous cell carcinomas. *Canc Biomarkers*: section A of Disease Markers. 2012;12(2):97–105.

[55] Yu CC, Hu FW, Ph DC, Chou MY. Targeting CD133 in the enhancement of chemosen- sitivity in oral squamous cell carcinomas-derived side population cancer stem cells. *Head Neck*. 2014.

[56] Clay MR, Tabor M, Owen JH, Carey TE, Bradford CR, Wolf GT, et al. Single-marker identification of head and neck squamous cell carcinoma cancer stem cells with aldehyde dehydrogenase. *Head Neck*. 2010;32(9):1195–201.

[57] Ginestier C, Hur MH, Charafe-Jauffret E, Monville F, Dutcher J, Brown M, et al. ALDH1 is a marker of normal and malignant human mammary stem cells and a predictor of poor clinical outcome. *Cell Stem Cell*. 2007;1(5):555–67.

[58] Charafe-Jauffret E, Ginestier C, Iovino F, Tarpin C, Diebel M, Esterni B, et al. Aldehyde dehydrogenase 1-positive cancer stem cells mediate metastasis and poor clinical outcome in inflammatory breast cancer. Clin Canc Res: an official journal of the American Associ- ation for Cancer Research. 2010;16(1):45–55.

[59] Krishnamurthy S, Dong Z, Vodopyanov D, Imai A, Helman JI, Prince ME, et al. Endothe- lial cell-initiated signaling promotes the survival and self-renewal of cancer stem cells. *Canc Res*. 2010;70(23):9969–78.

[60] Baumann P, Cremers N, Kroese F, Orend G, Chiquet-Ehrismann R, Uede T, et al. CD24 expression causes the acquisition of multiple cellular properties associated with tumor growth and metastasis. *Canc Res*. 2005;65(23):10783–93.

[61] Aigner S, Ramos CL, Hafezi-Moghadam A, Lawrence MB, Friederichs J, Altevogt P, et al. CD24 mediates rolling of breast carcinoma cells on P-selectin. *FASEB J*: official

publica- tion of the Federation of American Societies for Experimental Biology. 1998;12 (12):1241–51.

[62] Han J, Fujisawa T, Husain SR, Puri RK. Identification and characterization of cancer stem cells in human head and neck squamous cell carcinoma. *BMC Canc*. 2014;14:173.

[63] Lim SC, Oh SH. The role of CD24 in various human epithelial neoplasias. *Pathol Res Pract*. 2005;201(7):479–86.

[64] Fukusumi T, Ishii H, Konno M, Yasui, Nakahara S, Takenaka Y, et al. CD10 as a novel marker of therapeutic resistance and cancer stem cells in head and neck squamous cell carcinoma. *Brit J Canc*. 2014;111(3):506–14.

[65] Chen YC, Chen YW, Hsu HS, Tseng LM, Huang PI, Lu KH, et al. Aldehyde dehydroge- nase 1 is a putative marker for cancer stem cells in head and neck squamous cancer. *Biochem Biophys Res Commun*. 2009;385(3):307–13.

Chapter 5

Adult Acute Myeloid Leukemia – A Possible Relation to Disease Invasion and the Impact of Independent Prognostic Markers Associated with Survival Outcome

Mohamed El-Refaei and Fahd Al Qahtani

Additional information is available at the end of the chapter

http://dx.doi.org/10.5772/61179

Abstract

Over the past decade, leukemia exists and frequently occurs in adults. Radiation exposure, hereditary syndromes, smoking, age, and many other unknown factors are generally the major risk factors for leukemia. Acute myeloid leukemia (AML) is a hematological malignancy that is dispersed from its beginning and may be perceived as a prototype of metastatic cancer, yet leukemia is considered a highly malignant neoplasms responsible for a large number of cancer-related deaths. In addition, to uninhibited proliferation, leukemic cells dispense early from the bone marrow into the peripheral blood, followed by an infiltration of various organs such as lymph nodes, liver, spleen, lungs, intestinal tract, skin, or mucous membranes. Several studies are concerned with the critical role of angiogenesis in the development and growth of solid tumors and hematological malignancies. Moreover, angiogenic mediators created by AML cells act through external or internal autocrine loops, thereby directly indorsing cell survival, spread, and disease development. In recent years, many researchers focus on angiopioetins (Ang), an innovative family of angiogenic mediators, which have shown to be vital regulators of angiogenesis and vascular stability. Ang-1 and its antagonist Ang-2 act via the receptor tyrosine kinase sTie 2, which is expressed in endothelial cells (ECs) of the vasculature and in subset of hematopoietic stem cells. Binding of Ang-1 causes phosphorylation of sTie2 and ensures the integrity of the vasculature by stimulating interactions between ECs and endothelial support cells. This chapter reviews the incidence, mortality, pathogenesis, and diagnostic procedures of AML. As well as aims at evaluating serum levels of endostatin, MMP- 9, and uPAR in acute myeloid leukemia patients before chemotherapy and after achieving complete remission. At the same time, the chapter also assesses the pretreatment levels of plasma Ang-1, Ang-2, and sTie2, and the calculated ratio of Ang2/sTie2 receptor in a cohort of AML patients also studies their impact on the AML patients' overall survival.

Keywords: AML, endostatin, MMP- 9, uPAR, Angi-1, Angi-2, sTie2

1. Introduction

Cancer is considered as one of the major causes of mortality in the world. Despite the recent advances in science, cancer has not been cured yet [1]. Healthy cells are different from cancer cells. Cancer cells can do what others cells cannot such as: become resistant to growth inhibition; evade apoptosis; invade, metastasize, duplicate without limits; and support angiogenesis [2]. Cancer death rates remained approximately the same in the United States from 1975 through 2002, unlike heart disease. It is predicted that there will be about 15 million new cancer cases worldwide diagnosed and roughly 12 million cancer patients could die by 2020 [3].

Leukemia is a cancer of the body's blood-forming tissues. It's caused by the rapid production of abnormal white blood cells. The high number of abnormal white blood cells are not able to fight infection. The white blood cells can debilitate the ability of the bone marrow to produce red blood cells and platelets, figure 1 [4]. Leukemia develops when blood stem cells in the bone marrow change. The bone marrow will no longer grow and behave abnormally. The cells that are abnormal are called leukemia cells, figure 2. Leukemia cells will then start to crowd out the normal blood cells, causing the normal blood cells to not do their normal jobs over time [5].

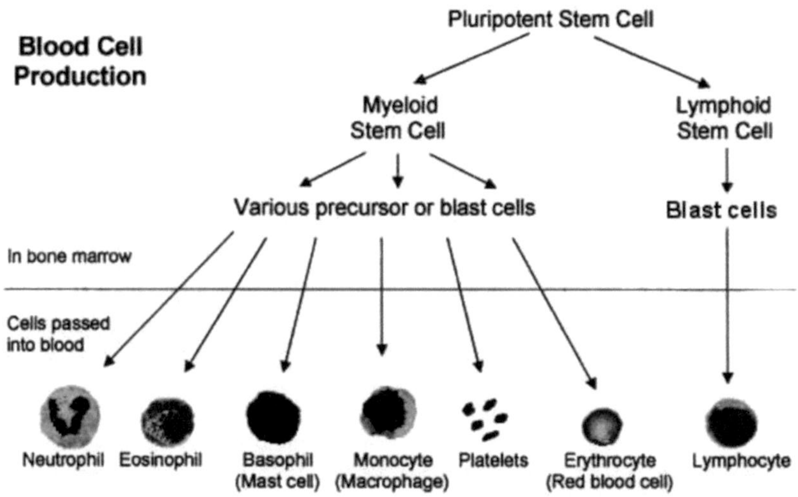

Figure 1. Stem cells and blood cell production.

There are many types of leukemia that exist. There are forms of leukemia that are more common in children, while other forms of leukemia only occur in adults. There are many types of risk factors for leukemia and they include, among others, age, hereditary syndromes, radiation exposure, smoking, and other unknown factors [6]. Furthermore, depending on the type of leukemia the signs and symptoms will vary. The type of blood that the stem cell leukemia develops determines the type of leukemia. Abnormal lymphoid stem cells develop lymphocytic leukemias, also known as lymphoblastic leukemias. Abnormal myeloid stem cells develop myelogenous leukemias [7, 8].

A genetically heterogeneous clonal disorder called acute myeloid leukemia (AML) is characterized by the accumulation of somatic genetic alterations in hematopoietic progenitor cells that transform mechanisms of self-renewal, differentiation, and proliferation [9]. Approximately 55% of adults with AML are detected by non-random clonal chromosome aberrations (i.e., balanced translocations, deletions, inversions, monosomies, and trisomies). These chromosome changes have been recognized as the most important prognostic factor of complete remission, risk of relapses, and long-term survival and have contributed to disease designation [10, 11]. A number of gene mutations and deregulated expression of genes have been identified in recent years, clarifying the immense heterogeneity of cytogenetically-defined AML subsets, especially the larger subsets of AML showing normal karyotype [12, 13].

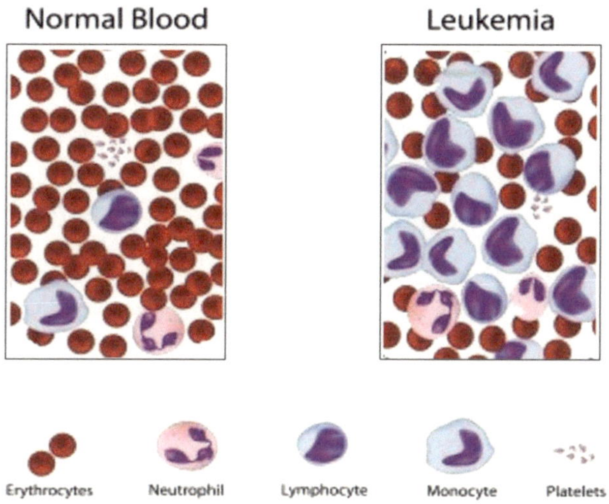

Figure 2. The normal and leukemic cells in the bone marrow.

Numerous studies have shown that angiogenesis is a crucial part in the growth and development of hematological malignancies and solid tumors [14]. Furthermore, there are several angiogenic mediators produced by AML cells that act through internal and external loops; thus promoting cell survival, spread of the disease, and proliferation [15]. It has been proven that basic fibroblast growth factor (b FGF) and vascular endothelial growth factor (VEGF) are major regulators of tumors with angiogenesis in AML; cellular VEGF represents an adverse prognostic factor [16].

In addition, many studies have focused on angiopoietins (Ang), which are a family of novel angiogenic mediators. Ang have been shown to be important regulators of angiogenesis and vascular stability [17]. Ang-1 and its antagonist, Ang-2, act through the tyrosine kinase sTie 2 receptor. These are expressed in endothelial cells (ECs) of the vasculature and in a subset of hematopoietic stem cells [18].

Acute leukemias are known to be a rare disease, but have a disproportionately large effect on cancer survival statistics [19]. They are the most common type of leukemia in adults, yet they continue to have the least survival rate of all other leukemias. Although, the rates have improved remarkably in the younger age groups, the prognosis in older patients continues to be very poor [20, 21].

2. Incidence and mortality

Incidence of acute leukemia accounts for <3% of all cancers. Leukemia constitutes as the leading cause of death due to cancer in children and persons<39 years old [22]. The most frequent form of leukemia is AML. AML accounts for about 25% of all leukemias in the Western world in adults [23]. U.S., Australia, and western Europe have the highest AML incidence worldwide [24]. AML in the U.S. during the years 1975–2003 was approximately 3.4 occurrences per 100,000 persons (= 2.5 per 100,000 persons when age-adjusted to the world standard population) [25].

The mortality associated with AML, just like its incidence, varies with factors such as age, gender, and race. The age-adjusted mortality rate in the U.S. seem to increase with age and peaks at 17.6 per 100,000 persons in people aging between 80 to 84. The age adjusted mortality rate for females in the years between 2000–2003 was 2.2 per 100,000, where it appears in 3.5 per 100,000 in males in the same period. Estimates show that approximately 7,800 adults will die annually of AML in the U.S. [26, 27]. However, an estimated 54,270 new cases of leukemia are expected in 2015 [28].

3. Etiology

Several risk factors have been associated with AML. Known risk factors only account for a small number of cases that were observed [29]. This will include age, antecedent hematologic disease, and genetic disorders, as well as exposures to chemical or other occupational hazards, radiation, viruses, chemical, and previous chemotherapy [30, 31]. There are several congenital conditions that may increase the risk of leukemia; the most common is most likely Down syndrome, which is associated with a 10- to 18-fold increase in the risk of AML [32].

4. Pathogenesis

A repercussion of specific chromosome translocations of the pathogenesis of AML are associated with the appearance of oncogenic fusion proteins. One of the fusion proteins is generally a transcription factor where the other partner is a variable in function and often involved in the control of apoptosis and cell survival. AML-associated fusion proteins function as aberrant transcriptional regulators that interfere with the process of myeloid differentiation, which determines the stage-specific arrest of maturation and enhance cell survival in a cell-type specific manner as a consequence [33].

The French-American-British (FAB) system (Table 1) described AML subtypes as M0 through M7. However, AML has been reclassified by the World Health Organization (WHO) into four categories in an attempt to predict the prognosis and biologic properties of AML subcategories more accurately and to enhance the clinical relevance of the system [34].

French - American - British classifications
M0: Myeloblastic without maturation
M1: Myeloblastic with minimal maturation
M2: Myeloblastic with maturation
M3: Promyelocytic; M3v: Promyelocytic ("microgranular")
M4: Myelomonocytic; M4 Eo: Myeloblastic with abnormal eosinophils (Eo)
M5: Monocytic: poorly (M5a) or well differentiated (M5b)
M6: Erythroleukemia
M7: Megakaryoblastic

Table 1. AML classification.

5. WHO classification

According to WHO, AML classifies depending on morphology, immunophenotype, genetics, and the combination of clinical features [35]. In the hopes that future work will elucidate molecular pathways that may be amenable to targeted therapies, the classification tries to identify biologic entities (Table 2) [36, 37]. The subgroup "AML with recurrent genetic abnormalities" amounts to some primary AML entities. "AML with t (8;21) (q22;q22); RUNX1-RUNX1T1" and "AML with inv (16) (p13. 1q22) or t (16;16) (p13. 1;q22); CBFB-MYH11" are considered as AML regardless of bone marrow blast counts. In "APL with t (15;17) (q22;q12); PML-RARA", RARA translocations with other partner genes are recognized separately. The former category "AML with 11q23 (MLL) abnormalities" was redefined as "AML with t (9;11) (p22;q23); MLLT3-MLL" and is now a unique entity; balanced translocations other than that involving MLLT3 should be specified in the diagnosis. Three new cytogenetically defined entities were incorporated: "AML with t (6;9) (p23;q34); DEK-NUP214"; "AML with inv (3) (q21q26. 2) or at (3;3) (q21; q26. 2); RPN1-EVI1"; and "AML (megakaryoblastic) with t (1; 22) (p13;q13); RBM15-MKL1", a rare leukemia most common in infants. Two new provisional entities defined by the presence of gene mutations were added, "AML with mutated NPM1 [nucleophosmin (nucleolarphosphoproteinB23, Numatrin)]" and "AML with mutated CEBPA[CCAAT/enhancer binding protein (C/EBP), alpha]". There is growing evidence that these two gene mutations represent primary genetic lesions (so-called class II mutations) that impair hematopoietic differentiation.

Categories
Acute myeloid leukemia with recurrent genetic abnormalities
AML with t (8;21) (q22;q22); *RUNX1-RUNX1T1*
AML with inv (16) (p13. 1q22) or t (16;16) (p13. 1;q22); *CBFB-MYH11*
APL with t (15;17) (q22;q12); *PML-RARA**
AML with t (9;11) (p22;q23); *MLLT3-MLL*†
AML with t (6;9) (p23;q34); *DEK-NUP214*
AML with inv(3)(q21q26.2) or t(3;3)(q21;q26.2); *RPN1-EVI1*
AML (megakaryoblastic) with t (1;22) (p13;q13); *RBM15-MKL1*
Provisional entity: AML with mutated NPM1
Provisional entity: AML with mutated CEBPA
Acute myeloid leukemia withmyelodysplasia-related changes‡
Therapy-relatedmyeloid neoplasms§
Acute myeloid leukemia, not otherwise specified (NOS)
Acute myeloid leukemia with minimal differentiation
Acute myeloid leukemia without maturation
Acute myeloid leukemia with maturation
Acute myelomonocytic leukemia
Acute monoblastic/monocytic leukemia
Acute erythroid leukemia
Pure erythroid leukemia
Erythroleukemia, erythroid/myeloid
Acute megakaryoblastic leukemia
Acute basophilic leukemia
Acute panmyelosis with myelofibrosis (syn.: acute myelofibrosis; acute myelosclerosis)
Myeloid sarcoma (syn.: extramedullary myeloid tumor; granulocytic sarcoma;chloroma)
Myeloid proliferations related to Down syndrome
Transient abnormal myelopoiesis (syn.: transient myeloproliferative disorder)
Myeloid leukemia associated with Down syndrome
Blastic plasmacytoid dendritic cell neoplasm
Acute leukemias of ambiguous lineage
Acute undifferentiated leukemia
Mixed phenotype acute leukemia with t(9;22)(q34;q11.2); *BCR-ABL1*
Mixed phenotype acute leukemia with t(v;11q23); *MLL* rearranged
Mixed phenotype acute leukemia, B/myeloid, NOS
Mixed phenotype acute leukemia, T/myeloid, NOS
Provisional entity: Natural killer(NK)–celllymphoblastic leukemia/lymphoma

Table 2. Acute myeloid leukemia and related precursor neoplasms and acute leukemias of ambiguous lineage (WHO).

6. Diagnostic procedures

6.1. Morphology

AML is first described by its morphology figure 3, or what the cancer cells look like when put under a microscope. The type of normal, immature white blood cell most closely resembles classified AML. The cancer that is in the cells that normally produce neutrophils is a subtype called myeloid leukemia in most patients with AML.

Using a May-Grunwald-Giemsa or a Wright-Giemsa stain, blood and marrow smears are morphologically examined.Using this method, they can give information about blood diseases (e.g., anemia, leukemia) that will change the aspect, leukocytes, number, size, or shape of erythrocytes and platelets [38]. 200 leukocytes on blood smears and 500 nucleated cells on marrow smears, with the latter containing spicules, is recommended to be counted. A marrow or blood blast count of 20% or more is required to be a diagnosis of AML, except for AML with t (8;21), t(15;17), t (16;16), or inv (16) and in a few cases of erythroleukemia. Included in the blast count are myeloblasts, monoblasts, and megakaryoblasts. AML with monoblasts, monocytic, or myelomonocytic differentiation and promonocytes, however, not abnormal monocytes are counted as blast equivalents. Only rare instances of pure erythroid leukemia can erythroblasts be not counted as blasts. Occasionally, the cytoplasm of the immature cells may contain abundant basophilic cytoplasm, containing variable numbers of indistinct coalescent granules. The diagnosis is M1 in case the immature cells are <10%, and the diagnosis will be AML-M2 if the immature cells are >10%. AML M2 baso showed a higher number of basophils along with the typical M2 morphology and was sometimes correlated with the t(6;9) [39].

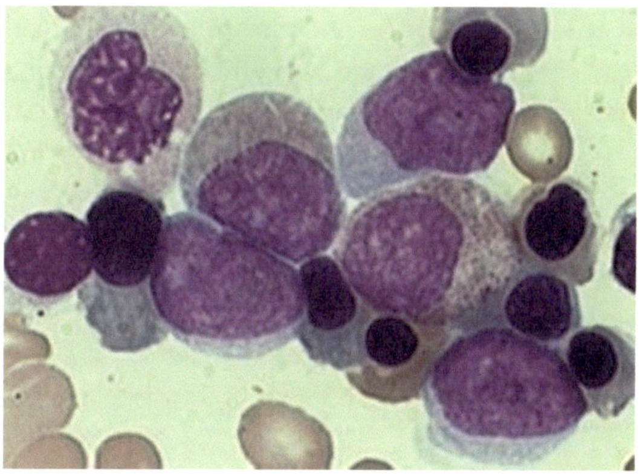

Figure 3. AML-M2 morphology. Note the presence of myeloid maturation.

6.2. Immunophenotyping

Immunophenotyping was performed by using a direct immunofluorescent technique and flow cytometry on peripheral blood specimens anti-coagulated by heparin of a newly diagnosed acute leukemia. For most markers, a commonly used criterion is 20% or more of leukemic cells expressing the marker [40], whereas for selected markers (e.g., cytoplasmic CD3, MPO, TdT, CD34, and CD117) a lower cutoff has been applied (10%). Phenotype acute leukemia (MPAL) diagnoses lineage assignment, and Measurement of Minimal Residual Disease is used to detect aberrant immunophenotypes (MRD), which is necessary for quantification of expression patterns of several surfaces and cytoplasmic antigens [41]. For morphological evaluation flow cytometry, determination of blast count should not be used as a substitute.

Immunophenotyping establishes the diagnosis of AML with minimal differentiation, acute megakaryoblastic leukemia, and acute leukemias of ambiguous lineage [42]. An AML with minimal differentiation is without morphologic and cytochemical evidence of myeloid differentiation [43].

Acute megakaryoblastic leukemia has 20% or more blasts, of which 50% or more are of megakaryocytic lineage; megakaryoblasts express less commonly CD42 one or more platelet glycoproteins CD41 and/or CD61. Acute Undifferentiated Leukemia (AUL) or those with blasts that express markers of more than one lineage (i.e., MPAL), are acute leukemias of ambiguous lineage, are rare leukemias, and comprise cases that show no evidence of lineage differing. AULs often express CD34 and/or CD38 and/or HLA-DR but lack lineage associated markers. Distinct blast populations or one blast population with markers of different lineages on the same cell or a combination of both can be contained in MPAL. WHO defines MPAL and encompasses subsets that are with or without genetic abnormalities [44].

6.3. Cytogenetic and molecular genetics

Chromosome preparation from peripheral blood and/or bone marrow was done according to standard techniques after culturing for 24 or 48 hours [45]. Colcemid treatment, hypotonic shock, and 3:1 methanol: acetic acid fixation and chromosome analysis were carried out on G-banded metaphase and were included in routine methods for metaphase spread preparations. According to the 1995 International System for Human Cytogenetic Nomenclature at least four metaphase were karyotyped and described [46]. In order to confirm or exclude the presence of leukemia-associated gene rearrangements, molecular genetic studies were performed. Thus, either fluorescence with LSI Dual Color Break Apart Rearrangement probe for Mixed Lineage Leukemia (MLL) or Reverse Transcriptase Polymerase Chain Reaction (RT-PCR) for detecting AML rearrangements were used [47].

6.4. Genome-wide studies

The major ways to distinguish AML subtypes involve hematopathologic diagnosis with flow cytometry and cytogenetic/molecular analyzes. Essential in the distinction among the sub-classes of AML is the notion that different subtypes of AML express different proteins, either at the cell surface, defining AML types distinguishable based on flow cytometry, or as a result of chromosomal rearrangements or gene mutations. Therefore, it is logical that a technique that can define a transcriptional gene expression globally should be able to distinguish among AML subtypes [48]. Identifiying novel genetic abnormalities and the promise of making the

http://dx.doi.org/10.5772/61179

systematic characterization of cancer genomes feasible has resulted in progress in genomics technology. For example, gene- and micro RNA-expression profiling have proven valuable for the discovery of novel leukemia subgroups and of prognostic signatures [49]. Uniparental disomy (UPD) is when a genome-wide single nucleotide polymorphism (SNP)–based mapping arrays, giving both copy number and allele-specific information, led to the identification of a novel mechanism involved in the pathogenesis of AML [50]. UPD is due to a mitotic recombination event and may render a cell homozygous for a pre-existing mutation positioned in the affected genomic region. The power of SNP genotyping as a tool for gene discovery is shown by several recent studies [51]. Hopefully, high-throughput DNA sequence analysis will become possible at an affordable cost, while analyses of genomic copy number will continue to be informative with regard to the selection of candidate leukemia genes. This may ultimately result in the development of comprehensive, disease- and allele-specific oncogene mutation profiling strategies [52].

6.5. Additional diagnostic tests

A patient with AML may need additional diagnostic tests and procedures that can confirm the diagnosis. Leukemia usually does not form tumors, so imaging tests are not used for diagnosis and are often used to check infections or other problems that may occur. X-rays routinely looks for suspected lung infection. Moreover, imaging in a few cases may be done to determine disease extent if it is thought to be spread beyond the bone marrow and blood.

6.5.1. Computed tomography (CT)

The computed tomography (CT) scan is usually needed if it is suspected that leukemia is growing in an organ, such as the spleen. Unlike a regular x-ray, CT scans can illustrate in detail soft tissues. In some cases, a CT scan can be used to guide the biopsy needle into areas of abnormality, such as an abscess [53].

6.5.2. Magnetic resonance imaging (MRI) scan

Asymptomatic patients are diagnosed with acute leukemia after the identification of abnormal peripheral blood counts. However, magnetic resonance imaging (MRI) has found that abnormal bone marrow signals appear in patients who have not been previously diagnosed with leukemia.The differentiation between benign marrow edema and tumorous involvement of the bone marrow is the measurement of the tissue microstructure the diffusion-weighted imaging reflects the random motion of water protons. MRI enables precise assessment of bone marrow infiltration early and before osteolytic changes become visible by conventional radiology imaging or CT scans [54].

6.5.3. Ultrasound

Ultrasound uses sound waves and ultrasound echoes and then produces a picture of internal organs or masses. Usually for this test, a small, microphone-like instrument called a transducer is placed on the skin. These transducers emit sound waves and pick up echoes as they bounce off organs in the body. The echos are then converted into an image that is displayed on a computer. Ultrasounds are used to look at the lymph nodes near the surface of the body or look at the enlarged organs inside the abdomen such as the kidneys, liver, and spleen [55].

7. Prognostic factors

The patient characteristics and general health condition of those related to characteristics particular to the AML clone are prognostic factors that may be subdivided. Patient characteristics and general health condition usually predict treatment-related mortality (TRM) and becomes important as patient age increases. Characteristics particular to the AML clone predicts resistance to at least conventional therapy. The following studies are aimed at assessing the pretreatment levels of plasma Ang-1, Ang-2, and sTie2, and the calculated ratio of Ang-2/sTie2 receptor in AML patients. Moreover, it aims to evaluate serum levels of endostatin, MMP- 9, and uPAR in AML patients before chemotherapy and after achieving complete remission. At the same time, it also studies the impact in the lives AML patients and their overall survival.

7.1. Circulating angiopoietin-2 is a strong prognostic factor in AML

The prognostic significance and over expression of cellular angiopoietin in the isolated peripheral AML blast and AML bone marrow is not demonstrable. Loges (2005) [56] showed that patients with high cellular Ang-2 had extended overall survival compared to those with low Ang-2 expression. Previously, we assessed the pretreatment levels of plasma Ang-1, Ang-2, and sTie2, and the calculated ratio of Ang-2/sTie2 receptor in a cohort of 71 AML patients in order to evaluate the impact in the lives of AML patients and their overall survival.

7.1.1. Materials

Seventy-one newly-diagnosed AML patients were tested in this study. Table 3 shows the patients' characteristics. All 71 patients were tested and followed up to 24 months (Table 3) or up until their deaths. Patients were followed in the oncology department at Mansoura Cancer Institute in Egypt where they were treated with approved protocols. 3+7 protocols (Daunorubicin 45 mg/m^2 iv days 1–3; Cytarabine 100 mg/m^2/day continuous infusion for 7 days) were used to treat the AML patients. Upon post remission, there was a high dose of cytarabine. Salvage therapy (HAM protocol) was applied (Cytarabine 3 gm/m^2 bid iv 3 hours infusion days 1–3; Mitoxantrone 10 mg/m^2 iv days 3–5) for patients who did not respond to the induction therapy. Complete hematological remission patients (bone marrow blast cells <5% in bone marrow) were submitted to consolidation therapy that contained a high dose cytrabine containint regimine (2 g/m^2/2hours/day × 4 days) + Daunorubicin 45 mg/m^2/day ×3 days. The M3 patients received all trans retinoic acid and went through chemotherapy. Nineteen normal, healthy subjects made up the normal control group.

Parameters	AML Patients
NO	71
Median age / years (range)	34 (16–55)
Male	40
Female	31
Mo	2
M1	12
M2	19
M3	3
M4	18
M5	10
M6	4
M7	3
Karyotypes	
Favorable; t(8:21), t(15-17), inv(16)	21
Intermediate; normal, +8, +22, others	41
Poor complex, –5, –7	9
Peripheral WBCs × 103/cmm	16.0 (9.5–89.2)
Peripheral blast cells %	20 (12.0–70.0)
Bone marrow Blast cells%; median(range)	55% (12–88%)
Follow up	24 months

Table 3. Patients' characteristics.

7.1.2. Methods

In a sterile tube with Ethylenediaminetetraacetic acid (EDTA), 6 ml of peripheral blood were collected from each AML patient at presentation and before the start of induction chemotherapy. For ten minutes in a refrigerated centrifuge, the plasma was separated by centrifugation at 1500 Xg. The separated plasma was reserved at -70ºC, thawed in use. Using commercially available kits from R&D systems (Minneapolis, MN, USA) and according to the manufacturer's instructions, Enzyme-linked immunosorbent assay (ELISA) were performed. Briefly, patient samples using the anticoagulant were collected with Ethylenediaminetetraacetic acid (EDTA) and stored at -80°C. Plasma samples were transferred to separate microplates, each containing a specific antibody for Ang-1, Ang-2, or sTie2. At room temperature, the mixtures were incubated for 2 hours. Plates were washed 4 times to remove unbound antigen. Enzyme-linked polyclonal antibodies specific for each angiogenic factor were then added, then incubated for 2 hours, followed by another washing step. At color development, adding of the substrate was stopped and a standard curve was used to compare the intensity of the color measure. Optical density of each well was determined at 570 nm.

7.1.3. Statistics

The software package SPSS version 10 has been used in this study. Mann-Whitney rank sum test for independent groups were used to analyze the differences in angiogenic factor level between AML and control groups. Furthermore, the Spearman rank correlation coefficient (Rs) was applied to assess the correlations between continuous variables. The Kaplan-Meier method was used for survival curves estimation. Overall, survival was the primary outcome of the studies and was calculated from the date of the first diagnosis to the death of the patient from any cause. In order to evaluate the predictive effect of each angiogenic factor, the univariate and multivariate Cox regression analysis was performed (figure 4, 5). Optimal cut-off points depend on 50 percentile of each angiogenic factor.

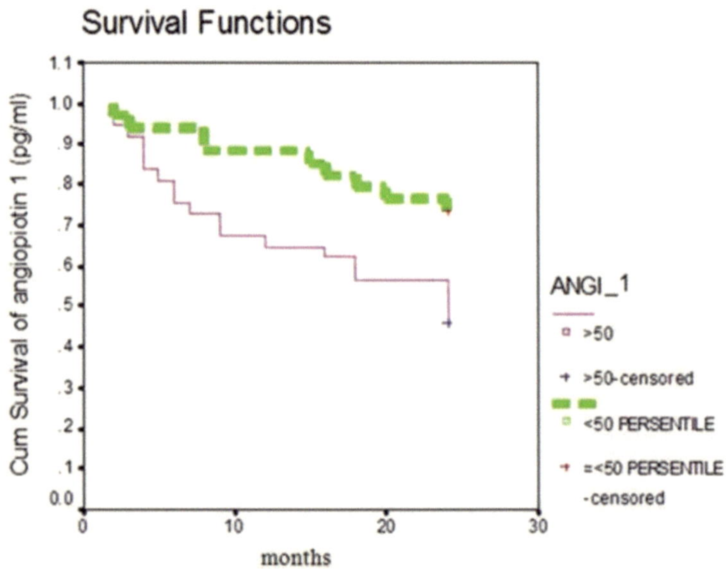

Figure 4. Kaplan-Meier survival analysis of AML patients according to Ang-1 levels. AML patients with high Ang-1 levels (≥260) displayed significantly poor survival rates than those with low Ang-1 levels (≤260) (P=0.018).

7.1.4. Results

7.1.4.1. Comparison of plasma levels of Ang-1, Ang-2, sTie2, and Ang-2/sTie2ratio in AML patients versus healthy controls

The plasma levels (median and range) of Ang-1, Ang-2, and sTie2 in pre-therapeutic AML patients and healthy volunteers are illustrated in Table 3. Circulating levels of Ang-2 and the calculated Ang-2/sTie2 ratio are decidedly higher in AML patients compared with controls

http://dx.doi.org/10.5772/61179

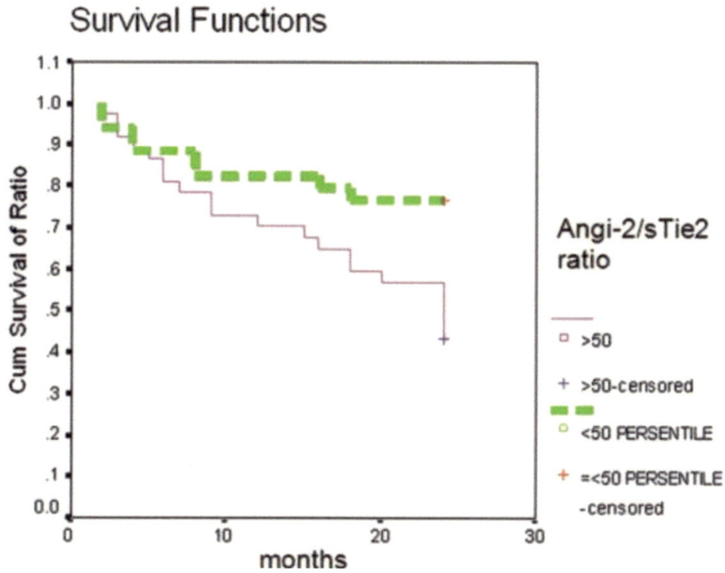

Figure 5. Kaplan-Meier survival analysis of AML patients according to Ang-2/sTie ratio. AML patients with a high Ang-2/sTie ratio (>279) displayed significantly poor survival rates than those with low Ang-2/sTie ratio (≤279) (P=0.004).

(P=0.002, P=0.015 respectively). In AML patients, the Ang-1 and sTie2 levels were not significantly compared with the controls (Table 4).

	Ang-1 (pg/ml)	Ang-2 (pg/ml)	sTie2 receptors ng/ml	Calculated Ang-2/sTie
Patients (n=71)	260(0–2250)	1400(133–4800)	3.9(1.0–35)	279 (32.4–1233)
Control (n=19)	180 (0–2195)	392 (185–1520)	3.1 (2–3.9)	139 (78–471)
P value	0.573	0.002**	0.057	0.015*

Table 4. Plasma angiopoietins levels in AML patients as compared to controls.

7.1.4.2. The association between plasma levels of Ang-1, Ang-2, sTie2, calculated Ang-2/sTie2 ratio, and clinico-pathological features

A significant correlation was obtained between Ang-2, determined Ang-2/sTie2 ratio, as well as patients' age with P value <0.05. On the other hand, no significant correlation was seen with sTie2 receptor that gives a P value of 0.786. Moreover, significant correlation was observed with Ang-2, sTie2, and WBCs with r=0.338, P=0.004, r=0.263, P=0.027. At the same time, no significant correlation has been seen in Ang-1 and calculated Ang-2/sTie2 ratio. The cell blast percentage in peripheral smears were significantly correlated to Ang-2 and sTie2 receptors with the following data obtained (r=0.365 P=0.002, r=0.387 P=0.001); no significant correlation with Ang-1 or Ang-2/sTie2 ratio (Table 5). Significant correlation appears clearly between LDH and Ang-1, Ang-2, and sTie2, contrary with Ang-2/sTie2 ratio. A positive correlation between

Ang-2 and Ang-2/sTie2 ratio with cytogenetic grades was found. On the other hand, a negative correlation was obtained with sTie2 receptor levels (P>0.1).

	Ang-1	Ang-2	sTie2 receptors	Ang-2/sTie2 ratio
Age (years)	0.254 0.030*	0.336 0.004*	-0.033 0.786	0.287 0.015*
WBCs (x10^3)	0.170 0.155	0.338 0.004*	0.263 0.027*	0.205 0.086
Peripheral blood	0.183 0.127	0.365 0.002*	0.387 0.001*	0.169 0.158
Blast in BM%	0.137 0.254	0.305 0.010*	0.317 0.007*	0.187 0.119
LDH	0.513 0.000*	0.362 0.002*	0.262 0.027	0.146 0.225
Cytogenetic	0. 258 0.030*	0.426 0.000*	0.170 0.157	0.333 0.005*

Table 5. Correlation angiopoietins and other prognostic markers.

7.1.4.3. Association between plasma levels of Ang-1, Ang-2, sTie2, calculated Ang-2/sTie2 ratio, and overall survival

In the study, univariate Cox proportional hazard analysis was dependent on 50% as a cutoff. This was done to assess the effect of circulating Ang-1, Ang-2, sTie2 levels, and Ang-2/sTie2 ratio on AML overall survival. The clinic-pathological variable as cytogenetic settled that a significant effect on the overall survival (p<0.005) variable as cytogenetic (intermediate vs. good vs. poor) and LDH (≤450 vs. >450).

AML survival was significantly associated with angiogenic factors Ang-1 (≤260 vs. >260), Ang-2 (≤1400 vs. >1400), Ang-2/sTie ratio (≤279 vs. >297) but sTie2 showed no effect. The death of Ang-2 was higher for the relative risk (RR) when the base line >1400 pg/ml (RR 5.7, with 95% confidence interval (CI))(0.061–0.50, p=0.001) had high significance with this ratio. CIs were 0.084–0.653, P=0.004 and the RR was 4.1 95%. No significant role of sTie2 >3.9 ng/ml (RR 1.24 95%, CI 0.481–3.220, p=0.652) table 6. Additionally, we performed multivariate Cox regression analysis incorporating all variables that were in significant effect on univariate analysis. The calculated Ang-2/sTie2 ratio was identified to be as the most prognostic factor with significant independent impact on survival (p = 0.000) (Table 7).

The findings from this study did not coordinate with Loges et al. (2005), wherein cellular Ang-2 was identified as the predictor of AML patients with favorable prognosis [56]. On the basis that the source of circulating Ang-2 from not only leukemic blasts, but also from other cell types such as endothelial cells [57,58], show the differences between soluble Ang-2 and cellular expression of Ang-2. Other hematological malignancies or solid tumors show limited studies considering prognostic relevance. Moreover, angiosarcoma [59], breast cancer [60], multiple myeloma, chronic myeloid leukemia [61], and recently in acute myeloid leukemia [58], higher levels of Ang-2 have been detected. An attractive therapeutic target when introducing anti-angiogenic strategies in the treatment of AML could be strategies in the treatment of AML for Ang-2.

http://dx.doi.org/10.5772/61179

Variable	No	RR(oddis ratio)	95%	P value
Age (years)				
≤ 25	33	0.894	0.346–2.311	0.817
≥ 25	38	1.12		
Sex				
Male	38	1.11	0.37–1.16	0.818
Female	33	0.88		
WBCS(x 10^3/l)				
≤ 16.2 x 10^3	36	0.104	0.034–0.320	0.000
> 16.2 x 10^3	35	3.62		
Bone Marrow				
infiltrate	38	0.202	0.073–0.561	0.002
≤ 50	33	4.95		
> 50				
Karyotype				
Good	21	2.34	1.11–4.17	0.014
Moderate	41	1.00	0.02–2.19	0.235
Poor	9	0.27		
LDH (U/L)				
≤ 450	36	0.143	0.049–0.417	0.0000
> 450	35	6.99		
Ang-1(pg/ml)				
260	34	0.306	0.113–0.831	0.0180
> 260	37	3.27		
Ang-2 (pg/ml)				
≤ 1400	34	0.177	0.061–0.510	0.001
> 1400	37	5.65		
S Tie				
receptor(ng/ml)	32	1.2	0.481–3.22	0.652
3.9	39	44.81		
> 3.9				
Ratio				
279	34	0.234	0.064–0.6530	0.004
> 279	37	4.27		0

Table 6. Univarate analysis of overall survival in AML patients.

95% confidence interval for B				
Model	**Lower bound**	**Upper bound**	**T**	**P**
Ang-1	0.000	0.000	-0.068	0.946
Ang-2	0.000	0.000	1.829	0.072
Ang-2/sTie ratio	-0.002	-0.001	-3.939	0.000**
WBCs	-0.007	0.002	-1.092	0.279
Peripheral Blast	-0.016	0.004	-1.266	0.210
Cell %	-0.010	0.008	-0.299	0.766
Blast in BM %	0.000	0.000	-0.732	0.467
LDH				

**Multivariate regression analysis of angiogenesis markers with other variants clarified that the ratio is the most foretelling predictor (p=0.000).

Table 7. Multivariate regression analysis of all variants.

Ang-2 blocks the therapeutic efficacy that has been manifested in solid tumors [62] and a recombinant Fc fusion protein against the action of angiopoietins is now being studied in a phase I study with patients that have advanced solid tumors. This study has concluded that the calculated ratio between Ang-2/sTie is a factor that should be a part of the decision-making process when choosing to use anti-angiogenic therapy.

7.2. Endostatin levels associated with favorable outcome

Inhibiting angiogenesis and tumor growth have been highly effective using endostatin [63, 64]. By inhibiting proliferation-inducing apoptosis in endothelial cells, it may mediate these biological effects [65]. Endostatin has been shown to induce regression of metastatic tumor in an animal model. The relation between endostatin levels and patients' outcome is scarce and the data surrounding endostatin levels in AML patients are controversial [66]. Tumor derived proteases generate the extracellular matrix protein collagen XVIII and is the C terminal anti-angiogenic fragment. It is not clear in AML patients the levels of prognostic relevance of serum endostatin. The study took serum levels of endostatin before chemotherapy and after complete remission in acute leukemia patients. The study also took the patients' outcome and correlated the endostatin levels.

7.2.1. Patients serum sample

Samples from 8 females and 22 males, with a median age of 37 within a range of 19 to 66 years old, with AML had been taken before chemotherapy. Also, 20 out of 30 patients were tested again once they were in complete remission (CR). From the healthy normal person group, ten samples were taken and matched with the same age and sex and were evaluated as the control group for reference. Enzyme linked immunosorbent assay (ELISA) were determined using serum endostatin (sE) levels.

7.3. Study results

7.3.1. Eendostatin levels in AML

In the control group, endostatin levels ranged from 5–20 ng/ml and have a median of 11.8 ng/ml. Pre-treatment serum endostatin (sE) levels ranged from 3–70 ng/ml and have a median of 14.8. The post-treatment sE levels ranged from 15.8–78 gm/ml with a median of 35 ng/ml figure 6. There was no statistically significant differences that were found between pre-treatment sE levels and normal controls. The post-treatment levels were statistically higher in pre-treatment controls. CR and sE and the relationship between them were then evaluated. Twenty out of the 30 AML patients reached CR. The patients who achieved CR had higher sE levels shown from the Wilcoxon tests.

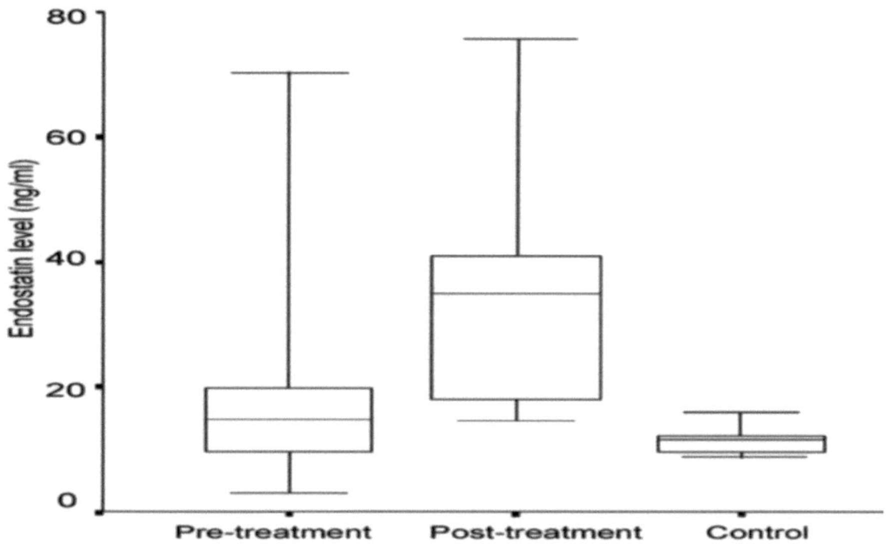

Figure 6. The Box-plot diagram showing the serum endostatin range levels in AML patients pre- and post-treatment compared with controls. Both 25th and 75th percentiles are illustrated with the upper and lower lines of each box. The median indicated with the line appears in each box. Pre-treatment compared to control (P>0.05); post treatment compared to control (P=0.000); and pre-treatment compared to post treatment (P= 0.001).

At the time of diagnosis as illustrated in Table 8, the sE levels increased markedly in the survived group when compared to those who died; the survived AML patients and control groups had a range of 9.6–70 ng/ml and median 38.15 compared with the levels of the died group that had a range of 3–25.5 ng/ml and median 14.8 (P= 0.04) and control group with a range 5–20 ng/ml and median 11.8 (P=0.026).

Group	Mean ± SD	Median	Range	P value
Died (n=19)	12.87± 6.07	14.5	(3-25.5)	
Survived (n=6)	56.58± 60.39	38.15	(9.6-70)	0.026
Control (n=10)	11.73± 4.28	11.8	(5-20)	

Table 8. Baseline serum endostatin levels in died AML patients as compared to the survived group as well as normal controls.

The baseline sElevel was not significantly correlated to age, hemoglobin level, peripheral WBCs counts, platelet counts, blast cells percentage in bone marrow, and BCDR (P>0.05) (Table 9).

Features	Endostatin	
	r	P
Age	0.166	0.444
Hemoglobin g/dl	0.068	0.745
WBCs× 10^3/cmm	0.112	0.593
Platelet count × 10^3/cmm	0.101	0.630
Bone Marrow Blast cell %	0.029	0.889
BCDR	- 0.01	0.98
BCDR (blast cell distribution ratio) = peripheral blast cell % / Bone marrow blast cell %		

Table 9. Correlation between baseline endostatin levels and some clinical and laboratory parameters.

The prognostic value of sE was then evaluated by dividing AML patients into low and high sE groups using the 75 percentile level of AML group (i.e., 20.5 ng/ml) as the cut off. As illustrated in Table 10 and Figure 7, high sE patients survived for a significantly longer time than low sE patients (P=0.02).

Endostatin level	Total	Died	% Censored	Mean Survival time	P value
Below 75%	19	17	10.53%	18.84	0.02
Above 75%	6	8	66.67%	36.33	

Table 10. Forty-eight weeks disease-free survival of the studied cases in relation to the pre-treatment serum endostatin level.

http://dx.doi.org/10.5772/61179

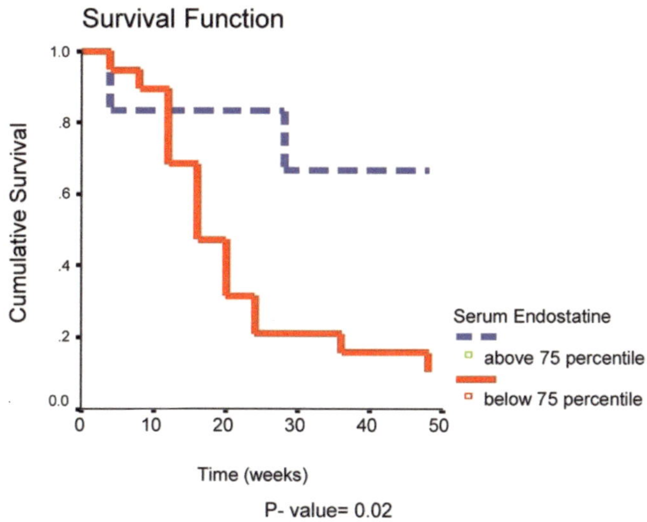

Figure 7. The overall survival of AML patients, according to pre-treatment concentrations of serum endostatin. The 75% concentration level of serum endostatin was used as cut off value.

The study showed that there was not much difference in the endostatin serum levels of the pre-treatment AML patients compared to the normal control group. The baseline for AML patients was lower than at CR. There was no correlation between pre-treatment endostatin levels, age, platelet counts, bone marrow blast cell counts, peripheral white blood cell counts, and blast cell distribution ratio. AML patients were divided into high and low sE groups using the 75 percentile of sE levels of the patient group and showed the prognostic value of sE. The study showed that the group with the high sE levels survived a longer time than the patients that had a low sE levels. The results conclude that the elevated endostatin levels in AML diagnosis is a good prognostic marker for patients' outcome. Wide-scale study is recommended in order to establish the clinical value of this study.

7.4. Role of metalloproteinase and urokinase in acute myeloid leukemia

An important role of the matrix metalloproteinase (MMPs) and urokinase may be important when trying to find tumor invasion and metastasis. An anchored membrane protein that promotes generation of plasmin on the surface of cell types is the Urokinase-type plasminogen activator receptor (uPAR-CD87), which is a glycosyl phosphatidyl inositol (GIP) and facilitates cellular tissue invasion and extravasation. Inflammatory cells or inaction of neoplastic promotes invasion from UPAR by proteolysis of urokinase [67, 68].

The collagens elastin and gelatin are a family of enzymes with the common ability to degrade various components of ECM [69]; they are also called MMPs. This family of enzymes all help the physiological processes that occur when the tissue is remodeling and repairing. The determination of these parameters in the blood are recommended as non-invasive tools in cancer diagnosis and monitoring may be reflected in body fluids called Cellular Concentration of MMPs [70].

Components of ECM, cytokines, hormones, growth factors, or a variety of biochemical stimuli all modulate the transcription of MMPs [71]. Various extracellular proteinases such as plasmin and urokinase are catalyzed by the activation of pro-MMP. Crucial roles of MMPs and soluble urokinase-type plasminogen activator receptor (suPAR) in the invasiveness of many malignant disorders have been accumulated in evidences from recent studies. The studies assessed the levels of MMP-9, uPAR in AML patients and compared them with previous clinicopathological status [72].

7.4.1. Methods and Patients

Twenty-five males and 18 females who were recently diagnosed with AML were used in the study. The ages ranged from 26 to 73 years old, with a mean of 46.8. The AML patients were studied at the time they were diagnosed, after starting chemotherapy, and during any relapses. During the induction of chemotherapy, seven patients died. The French-American-British (FAB) study group and immunophenotypic studies performed the diagnosis [73]. There were no patients that had a history of chemotherapy or radiotherapy that were diagnosed with hematological disorders. The criteria proposed by Cheson et al.[74] is the Morphologic CR. Peripheral blood counting was obtained through WBC and a percentage of blast cells. Blast cell distribution ratio (BCDR) was equal to the ratio between peripheral absolute blast cell counts to absolute bone marrow blast cell count.

The following FAB subtypes 2 M7, 4 M3, 4 M4, 4 M6, 6 M1, 7 M5, and 16 M2 were included in the AML patients. The normal subject group was made up of 10 normal subjects that matched the age and sex of the patients were used as the control group. A high-dose combination chemotherapy containing indarubicin, cytarabine, mitoxantrone, and etopside were treated in the AML patients. Remission induction therapy included one or two courses of cytarabine, etoposide, and idarubicin. The patients that achieved morphological CR received one course of intensive therapy with cytarabine and mitoxantrone. And lastly, all patients got consolidation treatments. All AML patients were then followed around for up to a year. EDTA tubes were used to collect blood samples and kept in ice before the plasma was separated.

The plasma was then removed within 2 hours by centrifugation for 30 minutes at 4°Celsius at 1800 g and stored frozen at -70°Celsius until the examination. Ficoll-Hypaque centrifugation was used to separate the mononuclear cell fraction. Most of the mononuclear cells in AML patients were blast cells that ranged from 0–96%. 1% Triton X-100 and protease inhibitors that were contained in cells were lysed in PBS. Lysates were centrifuged at 14,000 g for 10 minutes and 4°Celsius and the supernatants were stored at -70°Celsius until it was examined. The colorimetric assay kit determined the total protein. UPAR and ELISA were used to analyze the same amount of protein from each sample.

7.4.2. Immunophenotypic by flow cytometry

7.4.2.1. Preparation samples

Erythrocyte-lysed BM samples were used to diagnose all immunophenotyping study cases. A mircroscope adjusted to 1 x 10^6 in each tube quantified the number of cells. The following monoclonal antibodies were used to analyze antigen expression with fluorochrome-conjugated:

CD34

CD33

CD14

CD11b

CD45

CD10

CD19

CD22

CD3

CD5

CD7

Direct immunofluorescence was performed by first incubating 1 × 10^6 cells with the specific monoclonal antibody for 15 minutes in the dark at room temperature. To assess background fluorescence intensity, an isotype-matched negative control was used. Cells were lysed (FACS lysis solution) for 5 minutes and centrifuged at 250 g for 5 minutes. Before being re-suspended in PBS and examined, the cells were washed twice with phosphate-buffered saline (PBS). The EGIL recommendations were followed for immunologic criteria for lineage assignment [75].

7.4.2.2. Data analysis

EPICS flow cytometry was measured. For data acquisitions, the Cell quest software program was used. Over 10,000 events/tubes were measured..

Thresholds for positivity were based on isotype negative controls. Analytical gates were set on desired viable cells based on forward light scatter and side light scatter combined with exclusion of normal cells using a CD45 tube. The positivity threshold was 20% for all markers except for cytoplasmic or intra-nuclear antigens for which a 10% threshold was used [76].

7.4.2.3. Assay of suPAR and uPAR in cell lysates

As previously described [77], ELISA and suPAR were used. Immuno-plates were coated overnight with polyclonal antihuman uPAR antibodies. The wells were incubated with standard dilutions of purified recombinant suPAR or with 1:10 dilutions of plasma after blocking and washing. The volume equal to 20 ug of protein was put into each well for the cell lysates to determine protein concentrations. A mixture of monoclonal antihuman upper antibodies were rinsed and then incubated after antigen binding and then followed by alkaline phosphatase-conjugated antibodies. P-nitrophenyl phosphatase substrate was allowed to develop at room temperature to get a color reaction. Absorbance was read at 405 nm. The assay is 0.03 ng/ml lower detection limit. To estimate the total uPAR load in the cells in the circulation, the exact amount of uPAR in lysates was multiplied by the mononuclear cell count in the peripheral blood. This was tested without specific monoclonal antibodies.

7.4.2.4. Total MMP-9 enzyme-linked immunosorbent assay of plasma

Using a linked immunosorbent assay kit for human total MMP 9 according to the manual was used to determine total MMP-9 activities in the plasma. The diluted plasma samples or MMPs standards were mixed with 100 ul of 50 ul anti-MMP immunoglobulin G labeled with horseradish peroxidase in 10 mmol/l ethylenediaminetetra acetic acid. A 100-μl aliquot of the mixture was transferred to each well that was previously coated with an anti-MMP immunoglobulin G. The horseradish peroxidase-bound activity was detected by adding 100 μl volume of 0.15 mol/l citric acid sodium phosphate buffer at pH 4.9, containing 2.0 g/l of o-phenylenedianmine and 0.02% (v/v) hydrogen peroxide, followed by incubation at room temperature for 20 minutes. Adding 100 μl sulphuric acid 1 mol/l will stop the action. The micro-plate reader was adjusted to 492 nm for absorbance measurement. The human MMPs values were obtained from the standard curve.

7.4.3. Results

7.4.3.1. AML patients suPAR, cellular uPAR and MMP-9 levels versus control

At diagnosis the AML patients' suPAR and cellular PAR levels that were considered in mean were highly significant compared to the healthy controls with P=0.001 for both. However, during AML remission, the suPAR levels declined, achieving levels close to the control levels. On the contrary, during relapse, the levels increased again and came close to diagnosis levels (Table 11, Figure 8).

	suPAR (ng/ml)			cellular uPAR (ng/ mg protein/ 109 cells/l)			MMP-9 (ng/ml)
	At diagnosis	Remission	Replace		At diagnosis	Remission	Replace
AML patients	3.01±0.38	0.7±0.05	2.1±0.17	2.1± 0.17	11.21±1.71	44.5±0.76	13.56±1.07
Controls	1.02±0.14			0.26±0.02			42.05±2.18
P value	0.001	0.02	0.003	0.001	0.001	>0.05	0.001

Table 11. suPAR, cellular uPAR and MMP-9 in AML patients vs. controls.

http://dx.doi.org/10.5772/61179

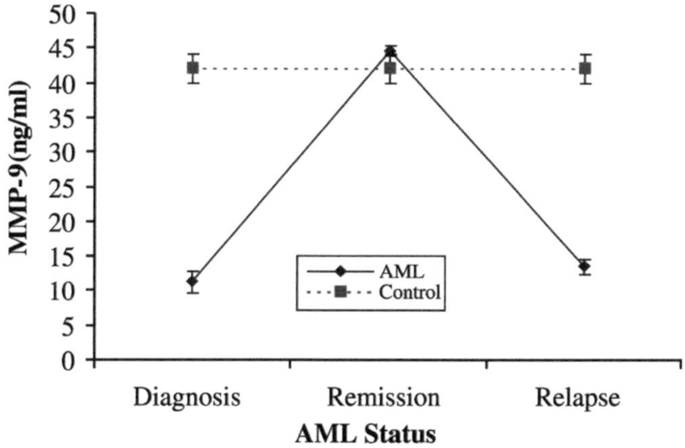

Figure 8. Soluble MMP-9 concentration levels at different AML status.

On the one hand, soluble MMP-9 levels were significantly lower in AML patients at diagnosis as compared to normal control, and elevated during AML remission and declined again during relapse (Table 11, Figure 9).

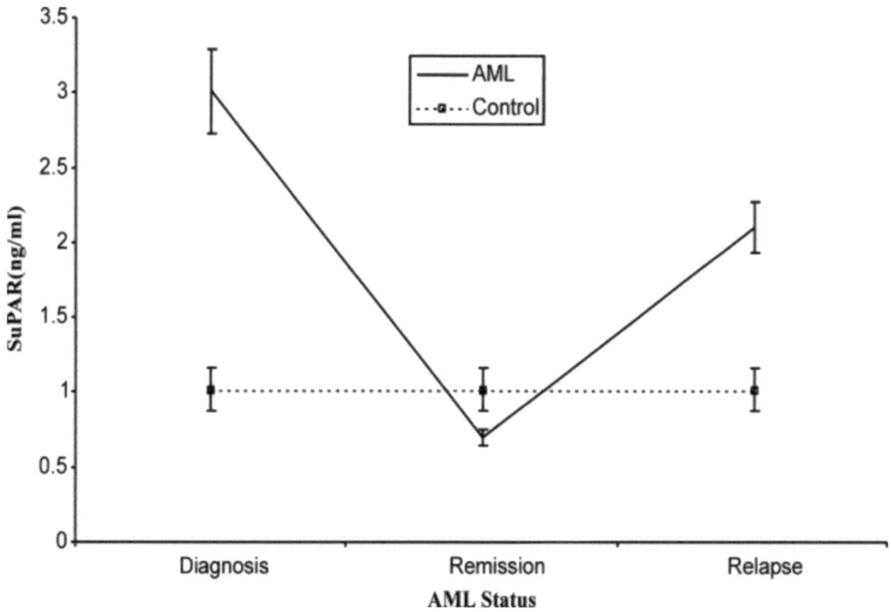

Figure 9. suPAR levels in different AML status.

On the other hand, AML patients who achieved complete induction remission have lower levels for both MMP-9 and suPAR as compared to patients who resist remission (P=0.001 for both, Table 12).

AML achieved remission	suPAR (ng/ml)	MMP-9(ng/ml)
Yes (27)	1.72±0.19	14.47±1.15
No (13)	3.27±0.20	34.02±5.2
P	0.001	0.001

Table 12. suPAR and MMP-9 levels at diagnosis in AML patients who achieved complete remission vs. who did not.

The levels of sMMP-9 and suPAR were significantly different according to AML status (Table 13). The MMP-9, cellular uPAR and suPAR diagnosis levels were uneven when classified according to FAB subtypes being highest among M5 (P<0.05 for all) (Tables 13 and 14).

suPAR (ng/ml)			MMP-9(ng/ml)		
Diagnosis	Remission	Relapse	Diagnosis	Remission	Relapse
(n=43)	(n= 36)	(n=10)	(n=43)	(n= 36)	(n=10)
3.01± 0.38	0.07±0.05	2.1±0.17	11.12±1.7	44.5±0.76	13.56±1.07

Table 13. suPAR and MMP-9 levels in different AML states.

	M1(n-6)	M2(n=6)	M3(n=4)	M4(n=4)	M5(n=7)	M6(n=4)	M7(n=2)	P
suPAR	1.9±0.01	3.31±0.57	2.1±0.43	3.6±0.41	5.3±0.4	0.85±0.4	0.80±0.1	0.03
cellular uPAR	0.33±0.1	0.8±0.15	0.4±0.11	0.96±0.14	1.26±0.21	0.53±0.1	0.11±0.11	<0.05
MMP-9	16.2±1.8	18.2±2.5	18.7±4.0	16.1±0.3	28.1±7.1	9.1±2.3	7.7±o.95	<0.05

Table 14. suPAR, cellular uPAR, MMP-9 levels in different FAB subtypes.

7.4.3.2. suPAR, MMP-9, and cellular uPAR levels and extramedullary involvement

In order to study whether MMP-9 and uPAR have significant effects in the AML blast cell invasion, the AML patient's serum levels of MMP-9, suPAR, and cellular uPAR were compared in the presence and absence of extramedullary involvement (Table 15). The AML subgroup with extramedullary involvement exhibit a significant elevation in MMP-9, cellular uPAR, and suPAR with a value P<0.05; P=0.001; 0.001, respectively.

7.4.3.3. Peripheral blast cells count, BCDR, cellular uPAR, suPAR, and MMP-9 correlation

A significant correlation was noticed between suPAR and MMP-9 and the peripheral blast cells counts (r=0.88; P=0.001; r=0.65; P=0.001), as well as BCDR (r=0.84; P=0.001; r=0.65; P=0.001). At the same time, there is a significant correlation between suPAR and cellular uPAR (r=0.88; P=0.001). Moreover, MMP-9 is correlated significantly with suPAR (r=0.84; p=0.001) as shown in Table 16.

	AML patients without extramedullary infiltration	AML patients with extramedullary infiltration	P value
suPAR (ng/ml)	4.48±0.65	1.94±0.31	0.001
Celluler uPAR (ng/mg protein/10^9/cells/1)	1.14±0.11	0.41±0.08	0.001
MMP-9 (ng/ml)	21.96±3.23	15.24±1.64	<0.05

Table 15. suPAR, cellular uPAR, and MMP-9 in AML patients with extramedullary infiltration vs. those without.

	Peripheral blast cells count	BCDR	cellular uPAR	MMP-9
suPAR	r = 0.881	r = 0.839	r = 0.881	r = 0.61
	p = 0.001	p = 0.001	p = 0.001	p = 0.001
MMP-9	r = 0.65	r = 0.65	r = 0.844	_
	p = 0.001	p = 0.001	p = 0.001	_

Table 16. Correlation between suPAR, MMP-9, and peripheral blast cells count, BCDR, and cellular uPAR.

The levels of suPAR, cellular uPAR, and MMP-9 at diagnosis were significantly higher in died AML patients group as compared to the survived group (Table 17).

	Survivors	Non-survivors	P value
suPAR	2.06 ± 0.17	7.86 ± 0.68	0.001
Cellular uPAR	0.54 vs. 0.07	1.61 ± 0.10	0.001
MMP-9	14.2 ± 0.96	37.87±4.47	0.001

Table 17. suPAR, cellular uPAR, and MMP-9 in AML survivors vs. AML non-survivors.

Elevated WBC count and suPAR levels had no correlation in a study in patients with chronic myeloid leukemia in chronic phase; it was also found that all suPAR levels in patient populations fell within the normal range. Moreover, it shows evidence that serum suPAR and MMP-9 are strong prognostic variables in AML patients. Levels were significantly higher in AML non-survivors when compared to AML survivors in super and mMP-9 diagnostic levels. suPAR and MMP-9 derived from AML blast cells could be a possible explanation for the prognostic value. suPAR and MMP-9 levels are higher in patients with extra-medullary infiltration according to the hypothesis. In conclusion, MMP-9 and suPAR levels might be used as a marker for disease activity and might contribute to blast cell dissemination. MMP-9 and suPAR may be target molecules in the strategy of treatmenting AML.

8. Treatment

AML has traditionally been considered a medical emergency, delaying induction chemotherapy until molecular testing results return; it may benefit some patients but harm others. Advanced age and adverse cytogenetics would show a lower CR rate and that risks associated with giving immediate intensive therapy to patients in whom poor prognostic characteristics with the risk of waiting to initiate treatment for additional test results to return [78]. Therapy for AML includes remission induction followed by post-remission chemotherapy for most patients. The aim of induction therapy in new patients diagnosed with AML is to lay down complete remission (CR), which in turn could optimize the cure and disease-free survival rate [79].

8.1. Remission induction therapy

The backbone of remission induction therapy consists of an anthracenedione or anthracycline combined with cytosine arabinoside (cytarabine, Ara-C), a regimen that has not changed since it was first introduced 30 years ago [80]. Daunorubicin is given at a dose of 45 $mg/m^2/d \times 3$ days, or mitoxantrone or idarubicin are given at doses of 12 $mg/m^2/d \times 3$ days in combination with cytarabine, which is administered as a continuous infusion at 100 or 200 $mg/m^2/d \times 7$ days (7+3 chemotherapy). Increasing the doses of cytarabine or the anthracycline, compares different anthracycliness or anthracenedione adding more drugs or using growth factors that prime agents or support care [81]; improved CR rates and disease-free survival commonly come at the price of increased treatment-related mortality than offsetting potential survival advantages. The median survival for older AML patients that follow these intensive approaches are typically 10 to 12 months, with higher median of survival for those entering CR, compared to non-responders or those achieving CR with incomplete platelet recovery (CRi).

8.2. Post-remission therapy

Usually, approaches to therapy for older AML patients who are in post-remission involve cytarabine and it is administered for a few days and then introduced in the remission setting. However, this is done alone or in combination with auntracene dione or antracycline for 1 to 2 cycles. Severe neurological toxicity in one-third of patients is associated with high doses of postremission cytrarbine. There is no added benefit to survival from more intense post-remission therapy or adding other agents. There is no added benefit from maintenance therapy through a more protracted course or post-remission therapy [82]. No randomized study shows that despite recommendations, no post-remission therapy or over post-remission therapy have any survival advanatages. Post-remission therapy that is becoming more common is Stem Cell Transplantation (SCT) is being considered more. SCT is done at the cost of high treatment mortality and offers the chance of a cure. SCTs have limited uses to the population and the limited matched donors who are related to patients have limited applicability. Ongoing non-myeloablative approaches studies have demonstrated the feasibility of more survival rates. Ablative approaches may not provide advantages over non-myeloabaltive regimens for older AML patients [83].

8.3. Role of transplantation

Although associated with an improved anti-leukemic effect compared with chemotherapy, the oral solution (OS) did not express consistently improve as shown from several prospective trials of evaluated autologous SCT. There remains a debate about what patients benefit from OS and in what type of patient an aggressive treatment should be reserved for and how SCT from a matched sibling donor has been part of standard care for 25 years [84]. Balancing the relapse risk that the patient faces with chemotherapy compared to the risk of the procedure itself is a decision that the patient faces. If a patient has a low relapse risk, they have a higher chance of responding if they relapse, so holding off on SCT to second CR is more practical. The risk factors that affect SCT could be influenced by many items such as the cytomegalovirus status of the donor and host, the age of the recipient and the donor, and the parity of a female donor. The degree of matching and the comorbidities present in the patient can be evaluated in a risk score [85]. A further complication in assessing the data for SCT in first CR is the method of assessment.

8.4. Molecular genetic implications for diagnosis and therapeutics

Molecular revelations have recently defined further prognostic cohorts. FMS-like tyrosine kinase 3 (FLT3) is important in the development of myeloid and lymphoid lineages may occur in 25% to 30% [86] for internal tandem duplications and domain or mutations of kinase activating loop. FLT3 ITD has proliferative advantage and anti-apoptotic signals and predicts shorter CR duration. FLT3-ITD to FLT3 wild-type has a high allele ratio and long length of duplication and location of insertion [87]. This information can help with the decision to go through allogeneic SCT even though the benefits may not be unanimous. FLT3 inhibitory activity has had little effect as monotherapy and at least three randomized trials are going in combination with chemo, which should also take account for molecular subsets. Fifty percent of cytogenetically normal acute myeloid leukemia (CN-AML) of the other intermediate group has nucleophosmin 1 (NPM1) mutations that result in delocalizing in the cytoplasm [88]. NPM1 mutations in the absence of FLT3-ITD are favorable outcomes that are similar to CBF leukemia in younger AML patients [89]. These types of patients can benefit from consolidated chemo and do not require CR after SCT. There are suggestions that NPM1 patients should receive additional all-trans-retinoic acid therapy, but this has not been proven. The prognostic value of the molecular biomarkers (e.g., NPM1) could be useful in predicting the outcome in older patients [90].

9. Conclusion and outcomes

AML in older adults is considered a difficult disease to be cured, representing one of the most challenging groups to be treated in oncology. However, advances in AML treatment have resulted in improved remission (an absence of signs and symptoms) and cure rates. This improvement may benefit treatment with intensive or alternative chemotherapy that is appropriate for the patient, enhanced by supportive performance status and cytogenetics.

Remission rates in adult AMLs are universally related to age, with an expected remission rate of more than 65% for those younger than 60 years. Earlier, the median survival of adult patients with AML at the beginning of treatment was 40 days. Recently, AML patients younger than 60 years have complete response rates of 70% to 80% after induction chemotherapy. Overall, survival is only about 50% for those who go into complete remission. Given the desperate nature of survival outcomes, clinical trials should be considered at diagnosis, along with considering the aggressiveness of therapy and patient-oriented treatment goals.

Acknowledgements

The authors wish to express their deepest gratitude to Professor Salah Aref, Hematology Department, Faculty of Medicine, Mansoura University, Egypt.

Author details

Mohamed El-Refaei[1,2*] and Fahd Al Qahtani[2]

*Address all correspondence to: melrefaei2000@yahoo.com

1 Molecular Biology Department, Genetic Engineering and Biotechnology Institute, Sadat City University, Egypt

2 Faculty of Medicine, AlBaha University, Kingdom of Saudi Arabia

References

[1] El-Refaei MF, El-Naa MM (2010) Inhibitory effect of caffeic acid phenethyl ester on mice bearing tumor involving angiostatic and apoptotic activities. Chemico-Biological Interactions. 186:152–156.

[2] Hanahan D, Weinberg RA (2000) The hallmarks of cancer. Cell J. 100(1):57–70.

[3] Bray F, Moller B (2006) Predicting the future burden of cancer. Nat Rev Can J. 6:63–74.

[4] Wade JC (2006) Viral infections in patients with hematological malignancies. Hematology Am SocHematolEduc Program. 368-374.

[5] Vardiman JW, Thiele J, Arber DA, Brunning RD, Borowitz MJ et al. (2009) The 2008 revision of the World Health Organization (WHO) classification of myeloid neoplasms and acute leukemia: Rationale and important changes. Blood. 114:937–951.

[6] Rosenberg PS, Wilson KL, Anderson WF (2012) Are incidence rates of adult leukemia in the United States significantly associated with birth cohort? Cancer Epidemiol Biomarkers Prev. (12):2159–66.

[7] Mauro MJ, Talpaz M, Radich JP (2013) Sequential therapy in chronic myelogenous leukemia: Where do emerging therapies fit within current treatment regimens. 11(11 Suppl 17):1–15.

[8] World Cancer Report (2014) World Health Organization. Chapter 5.13.

[9] Marcucci G, Haferlach T, Döhner H (2011) Molecular genetics of adult acute myeloid, leukemia, prognostic and therapeutic implications. Clin Oncol. 29(13):1798.

[10] Kurosawa S, Yamaguchi T, Miyawaki S, Uchida N, Sakura T et al. (2010) Prognostic factors and outcomes of adult patients with acute myeloid leukemia after first relapse. Haematologica. 95(11):1857–1864.

[11] Oriol A, Vives S, Hernández-Rivas J, Tormo M, Heras I (2009) Outcome after relapse of acute lymphoblastic leukemia in adult patients included in four consecutive risk-adapted trials by the PETHEMA Study Group. Haematologica. 95(4):589–96.

[12] Schlenk RF, Benner A, Hartmann V, Valle F, Weber C et al. (2003) Postremission therapy in acute myeloid leukemia: Results of the German multicenter AML HD93 treatment trial. Leukemia. 17:1521–1528.

[13] Bullinger L, Döhner K, Kranz R, Stirner C, Fröhling S (2008) An FLT3 gene-expression signature predicts clinical outcome in normal karyotype AML. Blood. 111(9): 4490–5.

[14] Ribatti D (2009) Is angiogenesis essential for the progression of hematological malignancies or is it an epiphenomenon? Leukemia. 23:433–434.

[15] Schliemann C, Bieker R, Thoennissen N, Gerss J, Liersch R et al. (2007) Circulating angiopoietin-2 is a strong prognostic factor in acute myeloid leukemia. Leukemia. 21:1901–1906.

[16] Loges S, Heil G, Bruweleit M, Schoder V, Butzal M (2005) Analysis of concerted expression of angiogenic growth factors in acute myeloid leukemia: Expression of angiopoietin-2 represents an independent prognostic factor for overall survival. American Society of Clinical Oncology. 23(6): 1109–1117.

[17] Qazi Y, MaddulaS, Balamurali K (2009) Ambati Mediators of ocular angiogenesis. J Genet. PMC. 88(4):495–515.

[18] Yuan HT, Khankin EV, Karumanchi SA, Parikh SM (2009) Angiopoietin 2 is a partial agonist/antagonist of Tie2 signaling in the endothelium. Mol Cell Biol. 8:2011–2022.

[19] Jemal A, Siegel R, Ward E, Murray T, Xu J et al. (2006) Cancer statistics. CA Cancer J Clin. 56:106–130.

[20] Redaelli A, Lee JM, Stephens JM, Pashos CL (2003) Epidemiology and clinical burden of acute myeloid leukemia. Expert Rev Anticancer Ther. 3:695–710.

[21] Sandler DP, Ross JA (1997) Epidemiology of acute leukemia in children and adults. Seminar Oncol. 24(1):3–16.

[22] Wingo PA, Cardinez CJ, Landis SH, Greenlee RT, Ries LA et al. (2003) Long-term trends in cancer mortality in the United States, 1930–1998. Cancer. 97(12 Suppl):3133–3275.

[23] RiesLAG HD, Krapcho M, Mariotto A et al. (2003) Cancer Statistics Review, 1975–2003. Bethesda, MD: National Cancer Institute. Based on November 2005 SEER data submission, posted to the SEER website, 2006.

[24] Jemal A, Thomas A, Murray T, Thun M (2002) Cancer statistics. CA Cancer J Clin. 52:23–47.

[25] Ries LAG EM, Kosary CL, Hankey BF et al. (2003) Cancer Statistics Review, 1975–2000. Bethesda, MD: National Cancer Institute. Available at URL: http://seer.cancer.Gov/csr/1975_2000 [accessed June 2004].

[26] American Cancer Society (2005) Cancer Facts and Figures Atlanta. American Cancer Society.

[27] Sekeres MA, Stone RM, Zahrieh D, Neuberg D, Morrison V et al. (2004) Decision-making and quality of life in older adults with acute myeloid leukemia or advanced myelodysplastic syndrome. Leukemia. 18:809–816.

[28] American Cancer Society (2015) Cancer Facts & Figures Atlanta: American Cancer Society.

[29] Sandler DP, Collman GW (1987) Cytogenetic and environmental factors in the etiology of the acute leukemias in adults. Am J Epidemiol. 126:1017–1032.

[30] Pogoda JM, Preston-Martin S, Nichols PW, Ross RK (2002) Smoking and risk of acute myeloid leukemia: results from a Los Angeles County case-control study. Am J Epidemiol.155:546–553.

[31] Pui CH (1995) Childhood leukemias. N Engl J Med. 332:1618–1630.

[32] Evans DI, Steward JK (1972) Down's syndrome and leukaemia. Lancet. 2(7790):1322.

[33] Alcalay M, Orleth A, Sebastiani C Meani N, Chiaradonna F et al. (2011) Common themes in the pathogenesis of acute myeloid leukemia. Oncogene. 20:5680–5694.

[34] Harris N, Jaffe E, Diebold J, Flandrin G, Muller-Hermelink HK et al. (1997) World Health Organization classification of neoplastic diseases of the hematopoietic and lymphoid tissues: Report of the Clinical Advisory. Committee meeting—Airlie House Virginia. J ClinOncol. 17:3835–3849.

[35] Vardiman JW, Thiele J, Arber DA, Brunning RD, Borowitz MJ et al. (2009) The 2008 revision of the World Health Organization (WHO) classification of myeloid neoplasms and acute leukemia: Rationale and important changes. Blood. 114:937.

[36] Swerdlow SH, Campo E, Harris NL, Jaffe ES, Pileri SA et al. (2008) WHO classification of tumors of hematopoietic and lymphoid tissues. Lyon France. IARC Press 439.

[37] Falini B, Tiacci E, Martelli MP, Ascani S, Pileri SA (2010) New classification of acute myeloid leukemia and precursor-related neoplasms: changes and unsolved issues. Discov Med. 10(53):281–92.

[38] Clark, G (2002) Staining procedures (1981), 4thed. Williams & Willkins. Krafts Woronzoff-Dashkoff, Kristine, Clinics in Laboratory Medicine. Vol 22.

[39] Pearson MG, Vardiman JW, Le Beau MM, Rowley JD, Schwartz S (1985) Increased numbers of marrow basophils may be associated with t(6:9) in ANLL. Am J Hematol. 18:393–403.

[40] Bain BJ, Barnett D, Linch D, Matutes E, Reilly JT (2002) Revised guideline on immunophenotyping in acute leukaemias and chronic lymphoproliferative disorders. Clin Lab Haematol. 24:1–13.

[41] Cherian S, Levin G, Yin Lo W, Mauck M, Kuhn D (2010) Evaluation of an 8-Color Flow Cytometric Reference Method for White Blood Cell Differential Enumeration. Cytometry Part B (Clinical Cytometry) 78B:319–328.

[42] Swerdlow SH, Campo E, Harris NL et al. (2008) WHO classification of tumours of hematopoietic and lymphoid tissues. Lyon, France: IARC Press.

[43] Bennet JM, Catovsky D, Daniel MT (1991) Proposal for the recognition of minimally differentiated acute myeloid leukaemia (AML-M0). Br J Haematol. 78(3):325-329.

[44] Döhner H, Estey EH, Amadori S, Appelbaum FR, Bu°chner T (2015) Diagnosis and management of acute myeloid leukemia in adults: Recommendations from an international expert panel, on behalf of the European Leukemia Net Bloom field 19 n30.

[45] Ritterbach J, Harbott J, Ritter J, Lampert F (1990) Chromosomal aberrations in childhood acute nonlymphoblastic leukemia. Haematol Blood Transfus. 33:153–156.

[46] Simons A, Shaffer LG, Hastings RJ (2013) Cytogenetic Nomenclature: Changes in the ISCN 2013 Compared to the 2009 Edition. Cytogenet Genome Res. [Epub ahead of print].

[47] Harbott J, Viehmann S, Borkhardt A, Henze G, Lampert F (1997) Incidence of TEL/AML1 fusion gene analyzed consecutively in children with acute lymphoblastic leukemia in relapse. Blood. 90:4933– 4937.

[48] Bacher U, Kohlmann A, Haferlach C, Haferlach T (2009) Gene expression profiling in acute myeloid leukaemia (AML). Best Pract Res ClinHaematol. 22:169–80.

[49] Wouters BJ, Lo°wenberg B, Delwel R (2009) A decade of genome-wide gene expression profiling in acute myeloid leukemia: Flashback and prospects. Blood. 113(2): 291-298.

[50] Marcucci G, Radmacher MD, Maharry K, Maharry K, Mrózek K et al. (2008). Micro RNA expression in cytogenetically normal acute myeloid leukemia. N Engl J Med. 358(18):1919–1928.

[51] Raghavan M, Lillington DM, Skoulakis S, Debernardi S, Chaplin T et al. (2005) Genome-wide single nucleotide polymorphism analysis reveals frequent partial uniparental disomy due to somatic recombination in acute myeloid leukemias. Cancer Res. 65(2):375–378.

[52] Mullighan CG, Miller CB, Radtke I, Phillips LA, Dalton J et al. (2008) BCR- ABL1 lymphoblastic leukaemia is characterized by the deletion of Ikaros. Nature. 453(7191):110–114.

[53] Owonikoko T, Agha M, Balassanian R, Smith R, Raptis A (2007) Gemtuzumab therapy for isolated extramedullary AML relapse following allogeneic stem-cell transplant. Nat ClinPractOncol. 4(8):491-5.

[54] El Rassi F, Little BP, Holloway S, Roberts D, Khoury HJ (2012) Early diagnosis of acute myeloid leukemia by computed tomography scan. American Society of Clinical Oncology.

[55] Xu ZF, Xu HX, Xie XY, Liu GJ, Zheng YL, Lu MD (2010) Renal cell carcinoma and renal angiomyolipoma: Differential diagnosis with real-time contrast-enhanced ultrasonography. J Ultrasound Med. 29(5):709–17.

[56] Loges S, Heil G, Bruweleit M, Schoder V, Butzal M, Fischer U et al. (2005) Analysis of concerted expression of angiogenic growth factors in acute myeloid leukemia: Expression of angiopoietin-2 represents an independent prognostic factor for overall survival. J ClinOncol. 23:1109–1117.

[57] Schliemann C, Bieker R, Thoennissen N, Gerss J, Liersch R et al. (2007) Circulating angiopoietin-2 is a strong prognostic factor in acute myeloid leukemia. Leukemia. 21:1901–1906.

[58] Schliemann C, Bieker R, Padro T, Kessler T, Hintelmann H et al. (2007) Expression of angiopoietins and their receptor Tie2 in the bone marrow of patients with acute myeloid leukemia. Haematologica. 91:1203–1211.

[59] Amo Y, Masuzawa M, Hamada Y, Katsuoka K (2004) Observations on angiopoietin 2 in patients with angiosarcoma. Sry Dermatol. 150:1028–1029.

[60] Cine GJ, Blann AD, Stonelake PS, Ryan P, Lip GY (2003) Plasma angiopoietin-1, angiopoietin-2 and Tie-2 in breast and prostate cancer: A comparison with VEGF and FIt-1. Eur J Clin Invest. 33:883–890.

[61] Quartarone E, Alonci A, Allegra A, Bellomo G, Calabro L, D'Angelo A et al. (2006) Differential levels of soluble angiopoietin-2 and Tie-2 in patients with haematological malignancies. Eur J Haematol. 77:480–485.

[62] Oliner J, Min H, Leal J, Yu D, Rao S et al. (2004) Suppression of angiogenesis and tumor growth by selective inhibition of angiopoitin-2. Cancer Cell. 6:507–516.

[63] Felbor U, Dreier L, Bryant RAR, Ploegh HL, Olsen BR, Mothes W (2000) Secreted cathepsin L generates endostatin from collagen XVIII. EMBO J. 19:1187–1194.

[64] Halfter W, Dong S, Schurer B, Cole GJ (1998) Collagen XVIII is a basement membrane heparan sulfate proteoglycan- can. J Biol Chem. 273(39):25404–25412.

[65] Dhanabal M, Ramchandran R, Waterman MJ, Lu H, Knebelmann B et al. (1999) Endostatin induces endothelial cell apoptosis. J Biol Chem. 274(17):11721–11726.

[66] Bajou K (2002) RoleofPAI-1plasminogen activator inhibitor intumor invasion and angiogenesis. Bull Mem Acad R Med Belg. 157(5–6):313–318.

[67] Zhao W, Wang X, Qu B, Huang X, Wang H (2002) Clinical significance of plasma tissue factor pathway and urokinase-type plasminogen activator system in cancer patients. Chin. Med. J. (Engl.). 115(5):702–704.

[68] Liotta LA, Tetler-Stevenson WG (1991) Tumor invasion and metastasis: An imbalance of positive and negative regulation. J Cancer Res. 51(Suppl. 18):5054s–5059s.

[69] Zucker S, Lysik RM, diMassimo BI, Zarrabi HM, Moll UM et al. (1995) Plasma assay of glatinase B: Tissue inhibitor of metalloproteinase complexes in cancer. Cancer. 76(4):700–708.

[70] Ries C, Petrides PE (1995) Cytokine regulation of matrixm metalloproteinase activity and its regulatory dysfunction in disease. BiolChem Hoppe-Seyler. 376(6):345–355.

[71] Tieghi A, Ciccone MB, ragotti ZL, cavazzini F, Porta MD (2003) Soluble urokinase-type plasminogen activator receptor (suPAR) as an independent factor predicting worse prognosis and extra-bone marrow involvement in multiple myeloma. Br J Hematol. 120(6):953–959.

[72] Bennett JM, Catovsky D, Daniel MTF landrin G, Galton DAG (1985) Proposed revised criteria for classification of acute myeloid leukemia. Are port of the French–American–British Cooperative Group. Ann Intern Med. 103(4):620–625.

[73] Cheson BD, Cassilteth PA, Head DR, Schiffer CA, Bennet JM (1990) Report ofthe National Cancer Institute-sponsored workshop on definitions of diagnosis and response in acute myeloid leukemia. J ClinOncol. 8 (5):813–819.

[74] Bene MC, Castoldi G, Knapp W, Ludwing WD, Matutes E et al. (1995) European Group for immunological classification of acute leukemias. Leukemia. 9 (10):1783–1786.

[75] Munoz L, Aveentin A, Villamor N, Junca J, Acebedo G et al. (2003) Immunophenotypic findings in acute leukemia with Flt3 internal Tandem duplication. Hematologica. 88(6):637–645.

[76] Stephens R, Pedersen W, Nielsen A, Hamers HJ, Hoyer-Hansen et al. (1997) ELISA determination of soluble urokinase receptor in blood from healthy donors and cancer patients. Clin Chem. 43(10):1868–1876.

[77] Sekeres MA (2008) Treatment of older adults with acute myeloid leukemia: State of the art and current perspectives. Haematologica. 93:1769–1772.

[78] Burnett AK, Hills RK, Milligan D, Goldstone AH, Prentice AG et al. (2010) Attempts to optimize induction and consolidation treatment in acute myeloid leukemia: Results of the MRCAML12 trial. J Clin Oncol. 28(4):586–595.

[79] Rai KR, Holland JF, Glidewell OJ, Weinberg V, Brunner K et al. (1981) Treatment of acute myelocytic leukemia: A study by cancer and leukemia group B. Blood. 58:1203–12.

[80] Rowe JM, Neuberg D, Friedenberg W, Bennett JM, Paietta E et al. (2004) A phase 3 study of three induction regimens and of priming with GM-CSF in older adults with acute myeloid leukemia: A trial by the Eastern Cooperative Oncology Group. Blood. 103:479–85.

[81] Stone RM, Berg DT, George SL, Dodge RK, Paciucci PA et al. (2001) Postremission therapy in older patients with de novo acute myeloid leukemia: A randomized trial comparing mitoxantrone and intermediate-dose cytarabine with standard-dose cytarabine. Blood. 98:548–53.

[82] Alyea EP, Kim HT, Ho V, Cutler C, Gribben J et al. (2005) Comparative outcome of nonmyeloablative and myeloablative allogeneic hematopoietic cell transplantation for patients older than 50 years of age. Blood 105:1810–4.

[83] Koreth J, Schlenk R, Kopecky KJ, Honda S, Sierra J et al. (2009) Allogeneic stem cell transplantation for acute myeloid leukemia in first complete remission: Systematic review and meta-analysis of prospective clinical trials. JAMA. 301:2349-2361.

[84] Gratwohl A, Stern M, Brand R, Apperley J, Baldomero H et al. (2009) European Group for Blood and Marrow Transplantation and the European Leukemia Net: Risk score for outcome after allogeneic hematopoietic stem cell transplantation: A retrospective analysis. Cancer. 115:4715–4726.

[85] Dohner H, Estey EH, Amadori S, Mead AJ, Burnett AK et al. (2010) Diagnosis and management of acute myeloid leukemia in adults: Recommendations from an international expert panel, on behalf of the European Leukemia Net. Blood. 115:453–474.

[86] Gale RE, Green C, Allen C, Mead AJ, Burnett AK et al. (2008) The impact of FLT3 internal tandem duplication mutant level, number, size, and interaction with NPM1

mutations in a large cohort of young adult patients with acute myeloid leukemia. Blood. 111:2776–2784.

[87] Falini B, Bolli N, Liso A, Martelli MP, Mannucci R et al. (2009) Altered nucleophosmin transport in acute myeloid leukaemia with mutated NPM1: Molecular basis and clinical implications. Leukemia. 23:1731–1743.

[88] Mrozek K, Marcucci G, Paschka P, Bloomfield CD (2008) Advances in molecular genetics and treatment of core-binding factor acute myeloid leukemia. Curr Opin Oncol. 20:711–718.

[89] Whitman SP, Maharry K, Radmacher MD, Becker H, Mrózek K et al. (2010) FLT3 internal tandem duplication associates with adverse outcome and gene- and micro RNAexpression signatures in patients 60 years of age or older with primary cytogenetically normal acute myeloid leukemia: A Cancer and Leukemia Group B study. Blood. 116:3622-3626.

Chapter 6

Pharmacological Inhibition of Intracellular Signaling Pathways in Radioresistant Anaplastic Thyroid Cancer

Dmitry Bulgin and Alexey Podcheko

Additional information is available at the end of the chapter

http://dx.doi.org/10.5772/62541

Abstract

Anaplastic thyroid cancer (ATC) is highly aggressive and has a poor therapeutic response and leads to high mortality. It has been shown that activation of intracellular c-Jun N-terminal kinase (JNK) and c-ABL signaling pathways is one of the manifestations of the highly resistant response to radiotherapy in ATC. Pharmacological inhibition of these pathways in combination with radiotherapy is a potential treatment modality of ATC.

Keywords: Anaplastic thyroid cancer, JNK signaling pathway, c-ABL signaling pathway, ionizing radiation, radioresistance, anthrapyrazolone, imatinib

1. Introduction

Thyroid malignant neoplasms are the most frequent endocrine tumor. They are classified into two categories, differentiated carcinoma and undifferentiated carcinoma (anaplastic carcinoma), based on the histological differentiation (Figure 1).

In the clinical course, differentiated thyroid carcinomas such as follicular cancer and papillary cancer have relatively good prognosis. ATC is among the most aggressive solid malignancies in human with a bad prognosis. In spite of active therapeutic and surgical treatment, ATC provides mean survival time less than 8 months after diagnosis [1]. ATC is widely metastatic, and it is highly resistant to regular therapeutic approaches such as surgical treatment, chemotherapy, or radiotherapy. It was confirmed that thyroid cells are relatively resistant to ionizing radiation (IR)-induced apoptosis [2, 3].

Currently, it is mainly approved that external beam radiotherapy of ATC should be combined with different anti-tumor pharmacological agents to have better local control of the tumor [4]. The main goal of this combination is to reduce the clonogenic capacity and radioresistance of

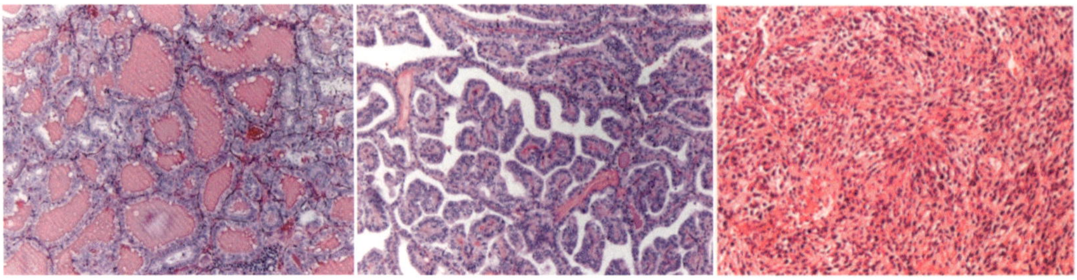

(a) (b) (c)

Figure 1. Thyroid malignant neoplasms histology: (a) follicular carcinoma; (b) papillary carcinoma; and (c) anaplastic carcinoma (courtesy of professor Masahiro Nakashima, Nagasaki University, Japan). Hematoxylin and eosin stain. Original magnification ×100.

ATC cells with the aim of further improving the radiotherapy effect. It is conceivably that molecular-targeted pharmacological agents can decrease cancer resistance to radiotherapy through modulation of DNA repair, cell death pathway, intracellular signal transduction [5, 6], or senescence-like terminal growth arrest [7].

2. Radiation therapy

Radiation therapy, like most anti-tumor treatments, achieves its therapeutic effect by inducing different types of cell death in tumors [8]. Over the past decade, our knowledge is rapidly increasing regarding the discovery of various molecular pathways involved in determining cell death after IR exposure [9]. The biological target of IR in the cell is DNA (Figure 2).

Double-strand breaks (DSBs) are the most destructive DNA alterations, which, if left unrepaired, may have serious consequences for cell survival, as they lead to genomic instability, chromosome aberrations, or cell death. DSBs are irreparable and more responsible than the single-strand DNA breaks for most of cell death in tumor as well as surrounding normal cells. Cells respond to DNA damage by activating complex processes at the level of molecules and genes to detect and repair DNA alterations. The formation of DSBs activated phosphorylation of H2AX (the subtype of histone H2A). The phosphorylated form of H2AX is called γ-H2AX [10]. Phosphorylation of H2AX plays a key role in DNA reparation, and it is necessary for the assembly of DNA repair molecules at the sites containing damaged chromatin as well as for activation of checkpoint proteins, which arrest the cell cycle progression [11]. The evaluation of γ-H2AX levels may allow not only to control the efficiency of anti-tumor therapy but also to predict cancer cell sensitivity to DNA-damaging anti-tumor agents and toxicity of anti-tumor treatment toward normal cells. It is possible to detect H2AX phosphorylation by specific γ-H2AX antibody and thus to detect DNA damage and repair *in situ* in individual cells. The presence of γ-H2AX in chromatin can be exposed shortly after induction of DSBs in the form of discrete nuclear foci (Figure 3) [12]. The presence of γ-H2AX-containing nuclear foci can be measured by microscopy, flow cytometry, and Western blotting of tissue/cell lysates [13].

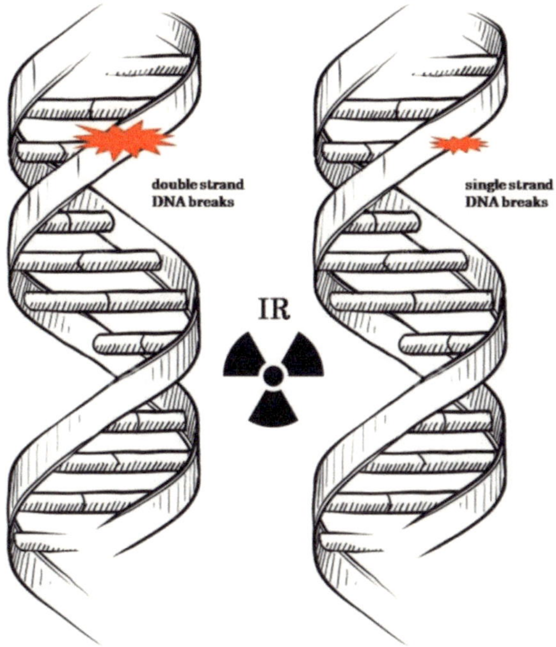

Figure 2. The biological target of IR in the cell is DNA. IR-induced DNA damage of cancer cells can lead to cell death.

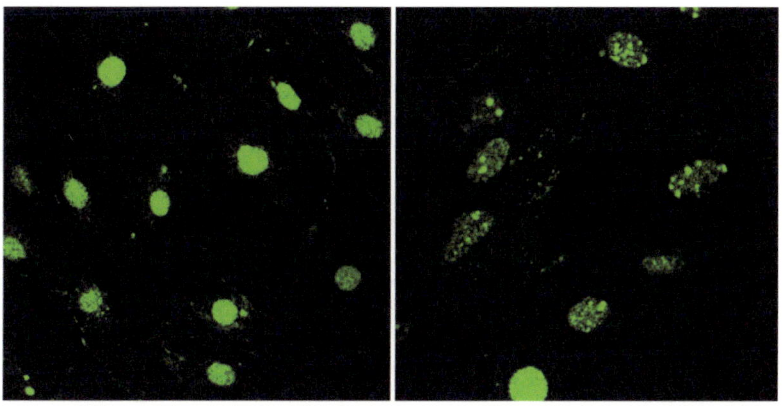

(a) (b)

Figure 3. IR induces γ-H2AX nuclear foci formation in ATC cell lines: (a) non-radiated; (b) in 24 hours after 10 Gy IR treatment (EXS-300 X-irradiator, Toshiba, Tokyo, Japan; 200 kV, 15 mA, 0.83 Gy/min). Compared to alternative methods of DNA damage assessment, the immunocytochemical approach is less cumbersome and offers much greater sensitivity. Fluorescent immunocytochemistry. Confocal fluorescent microscopy. Original magnification ×400.

The main goal of radiotherapy is to deprive tumor cells of their multiplication potential and finally to destroy the cancer cells. After IR exposure, cell death may occur by one or more of the following mechanisms: immediate or delayed apoptosis, mitotic-linked death (mitotic catastrophe), autophagy, and terminal growth arrest (senescence) associated with necrosis (Figure 4).

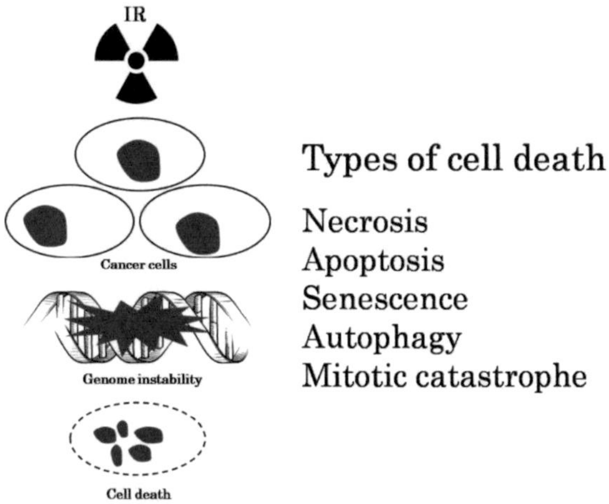

Figure 4. Mechanisms of cancer cell death triggered by IR.

Radiotherapy does not destroy cancer cells right away. It takes hours, days, or weeks of anti-tumor therapy before cancer cells start to die after which cancer cells continue dying for weeks to months after ending of radiotherapy. The efficiency of radiotherapy has much to gain by understanding the cell death mechanisms that are induced in tumor cells following irradiation (Table 1). Strategies to use specific pharmacological agents that can inhibit the activity of key molecules in intracellular signaling pathways combined with IR might potentiate therapy and enhance tumor cell death [14].

Types of cell death	Definition and characteristics	Associated changes	Detection methods
Necrosis	Cells visibly swell with breakdown of cell membrane. Typical nuclei with vacuolization and disintegrated cell organelles.	Sometimes not considered genetically determined. Drop of ATP levels. ROS over-generation.	Early permeability to vital dyes. Staining with propidium iodide. Electron microscopy.
Apoptosis	Programmed cell death. Cells shrink with blebbing of cell membranes. Condensed chromatin and DNA fragmentation.	Stimulated by cyclin D1 activation and by Myc. Can be inhibited by loss of wild-type p53. Caspase activation.	Sub-G1 peak in flow cytometry. Annexin-V staining. Quantification of $\Delta\Psi m$. Internucleosomal laddering.

Types of cell death	Definition and characteristics	Associated changes	Detection methods
		Dissipation of mitochondrial transmembrane potential ($\Delta\Psi m$).	
Senescence	Cells do not divide, although they remain metabolically active. Large and flat cells with increased granularity.	Stimulated by Ras mutations and telomerase shortening. Inhibited by the loss of wild-type p53, p16, and $p21^{WAF1}$.	Staining for β-galactosidase at pH 6 (SA-β-Gal+). Absence of DNA synthesis (BrdU incorporation).
Autophagy	Programmed cell death in which the cell digests itself. Formation of vacuoles in cytoplasm.	Cell death is accompanied by massive autophagic vacuolization of cytoplasm without condensation. LC3-I to LC3-II conversion (LC3, microtubule-associated protein).	Immunoblotting with LC3-specific antibodies. Immunofluorescence microscopy (LC3-GFP fusion protein).
Mitotic catastrophe	Cell death occurring during or after a faulty mitosis. Giant cells with two or more nuclei and partially condensed chromatin. Can lead to necrosis or apoptosis-like death (p53-independent).	Stimulated by deficiencies in proteins involved in G1 and G2 checkpoints and in mitotic spindle assembly. Can follow caspase-dependent or caspase-independent pathways.	Cells with two or more nuclei detected by microscopy or laser scanning cytometry. Aberrant mitotic figures. Accumulation in G2/M and polyploidy.

Table 1. Anti-proliferative response and cell death pathways observed upon radiotherapy.

3. JNK signaling pathway

c-Jun N-terminal kinases (JNKs) are multifunctional kinases, also known as stress-activated protein kinases be a part of superfamily of mitogen-activated protein kinases (MAPKs) that are involved in many physiological and pathological processes (Figure 5). At first, the JNKs were originally identified as ultraviolet-responsive protein kinases by their capacity to phosphorylate the N-terminal of the transcription factor c-Jun and by their activation in response to various stresses [15]. Initial research works have shown that JNKs can be triggered by various stimuli including growth factors [16, 17], cytokines [18], and stress factors [19]. It was demonstrated that IR with level of 10 Gy induced JNK activation with a maximum at 30 minutes and return to baseline at 12 hours after exposure in ATC cell lines [7].

Other observations have demonstrated the crucial role of JNK pathway in mediating apoptotic signaling in many cell death paradigms [20]. JNK signal transduction pathway regulates the cellular reaction to IR and activating radiation-induced apoptosis [21]. However, it was shown

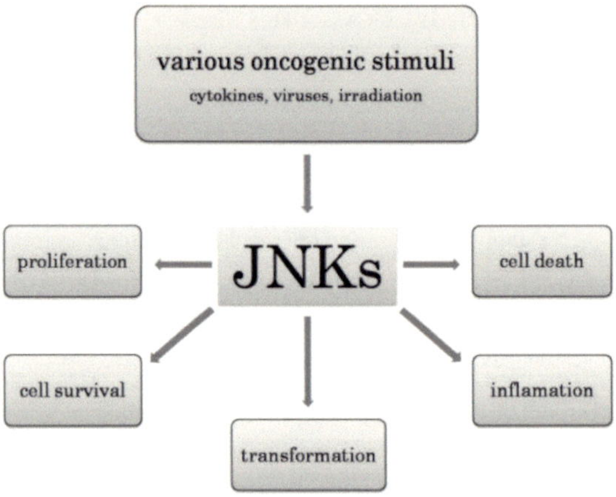

Figure 5. Various extracellular and intracellular stimuli can activate JNKs. Constant JNK activation influences tumourigenesis by both transcription-independent and transcription-dependent mechanisms involved in cell transformation, proliferation, survival, migration, suppression of cell death, and inflammatory processes in tumor.

that JNK cascade, via the stimulation of c-Jun and ATF-2 transcription factors, may provide DNA repair and cell survival (Figure 6) [22].

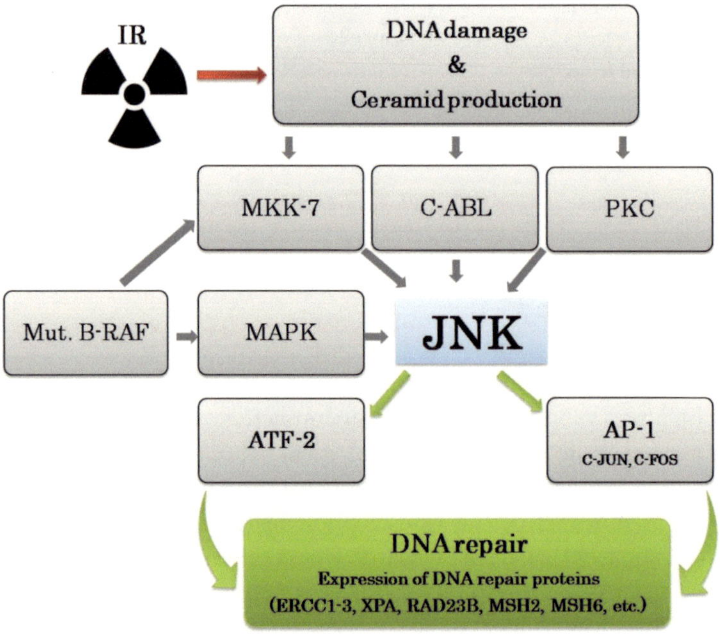

Figure 6. Role of JNK kinase in DNA repair after IR-induced extensive damage.

For that reason, it was proposed that JNK pathway inhibition could result in sensitization of distinct types of tumor cells to DNA damage.

http://dx.doi.org/10.5772/62541

4. c-ABL tyrosine kinase signaling pathway

c-ABL is an ubiquitously expressed tyrosine kinase that involves in various cellular signaling processes. The c-ABL is highly expressed in normal and cancer cells [23, 24]. c-ABL is frequently overexpressed in ATC cell lines (Figure 7) and thyroid cancer tissue samples (Figure 8).

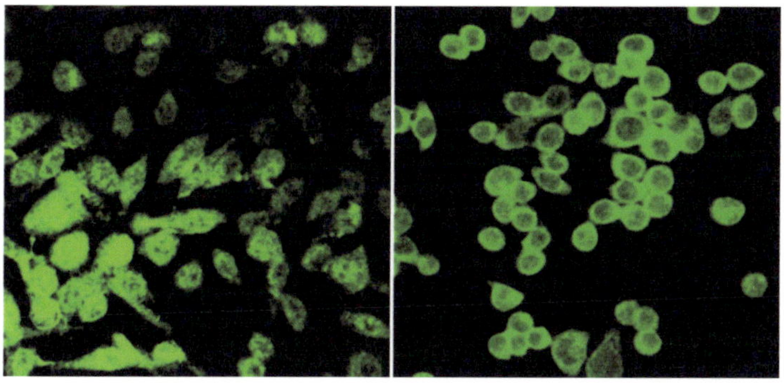

(a) (b)

Figure 7. c-ABL expression in ATC cell lines: (a) FRO cell line and (b) ARO cell line. Fluorescent immunocytochemistry. Confocal fluorescent microscopy. Original magnification ×400.

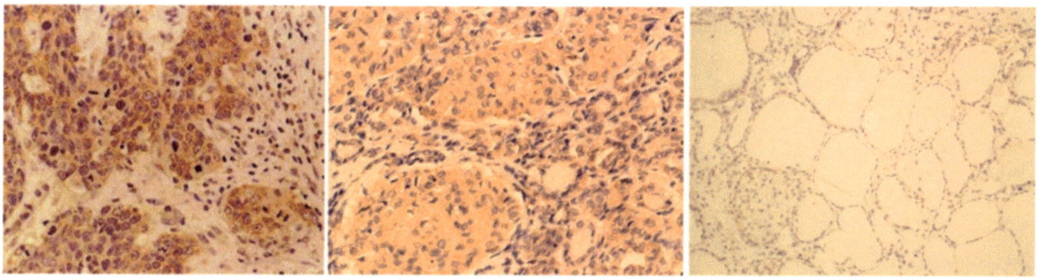

(a) (b) (c)

Figure 8. The different expression pattern of c-ABL: (a) high level of expression of c-ABL in anaplastic thyroid carcinoma; (b) follicular carcinoma; and (c) goiter. Immunohistochemistry: antibodies used were anti-c-ABL. Original magnification ×200 (a,b) and ×100 (c).

Previous experiments indicated that c-ABL is involved in regulation of the cell cycle and the cellular genotoxic stress response pathways. It was demonstrated that the growth arrest was accompanied by the down-regulation of c-ABL phosphorylation and of cyclins A and B1 levels and by the up-regulation of the cell cycle inhibitor $p21^{cip1}$. Also, it was presented that $p21^{cip1}$ expression is associated with improved survival in patients after adjuvant radiotherapy [25]. The cellular reaction elicited by c-ABL depends upon its location in cells. Accumulation of c-ABL in the cytoplasm results in cell survival and proliferation. By contrast, nuclear c-ABL becomes activated and induces apoptosis following genotoxic stress [26]. DNA damage caused by IR and other DNA-damaging agents has been shown to result in activation of the c-ABL (Figure 9) [27].

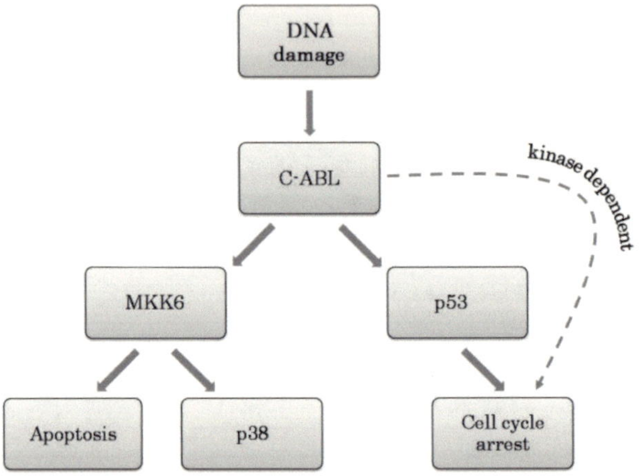

Figure 9. Nuclear targeting of c-ABL in response to DNA damage.

It was demonstrated that IR induces redistribution of c-ABL between nucleus and cytoplasm in ATC cells (Figure 10) [28].

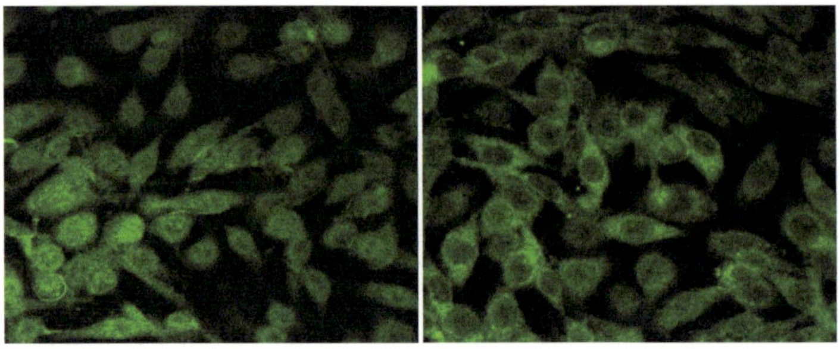

(a) (b)

Figure 10. IR induces redistribution of c-ABL between nucleus and cytoplasm in ATC cells. Translocation of c-ABL in FRO cells after IR treatment (EXS-300 X-irradiator, Toshiba, Tokyo, Japan; 200 kV, 15 mA, 0.83 Gy/min): (a) non-radiated; (b) in 6 hours after 10 Gy IR treatment. Fluorescent immunocytochemistry. Confocal fluorescent microscopy. Original magnification ×400.

Notably, nuclear targeting of c-ABL is required for the induction of apoptosis in response to DNA damage. Overexpression of c-ABL activates cell cycle arrest in G1, which requires kinase activity and nuclear localizing signals and depends on the wild-type p53 tumor suppressor (Figure 10). In addition, c-ABL binds p53 and enhances the DNA binding and transcriptional activity of p53 [29, 30].

Previous studies have revealed that loss of wild-type p53 function by mutation of the gene can lead differentiated thyroid cancer to anaplastic change [31, 32]. ATC is harbor mutations of p53 in 80–90% of cases and characterized by aggressive course of disease. It was previously demonstrated that thyroid cancer cells with p53 mutation are relatively resistant to IR-induced apoptosis [33]. Relationships between c-ABL and p53 revealed dependence of p53-deficient cells from c-ABL for enhanced proliferation, suggesting that pharmacologic inhibition of c-ABL may have therapeutic value in the p53-deficient cancer cells [34]. Hence, pharmacological inhibition of c-ABL kinase activity can modify the response of ATC cells to IR and could be a promising treatment modality.

5. Senescence-like terminal growth arrest

Senescence is a physiological process of changes in cell metabolism associated with a series of inductive, permissive, and restrictive communications that limit the cell proliferative capacity. Senescent cells are viable but non-dividing, stop to synthesize DNA, and become enlarged and flattened with an increased granularity. Recent data show that senescence may act as an acute, drug- or IR-induced growth arrest program in numerous stromal and epithelial tumors [35]. It was found that IR induces senescence-like phenotype (SLP) associated with terminal growth arrest in ATC cell lines and also in primary thyrocyte line in time- and dose-dependent manner [36].

The induction of SLP in thyroid cells can be identified by the following:

- Senescence-associated β-galactosidase (SA-β-Gal) staining method (Figure 11)
- Dual-flow cytometric analysis of cell proliferation and side light scatter using vital staining with PKH-2 dye
- Double labeling technique for SA-β-Gal and 5-bromo-2′-deoxyuridine (BrdU)
- Staining for SA-β-Gal with consequent anti-thyroglobulin immunocytochemistry (Figure 12)

6. Anthrapyrazolone as a specific inhibitor of JNK signaling pathway

Anthrapyrazolone is a synthetic polyaromatic small molecule–specific inhibitor of c-JNK signaling (Figure 13). Anthrapyrazolone acts as a reversible ATP-competitive inhibitor with an identical capability toward JNK1, JNK2, and JNK3 with >20-fold selectivity versus various tested kinases other than JNKs [37, 38].

In cell cultures, anthrapyrazolone shows dose-dependent inhibition of c-Jun phosphorylation in the range of 5–50 μM [38]. It was demonstrated that combination of anthrapyrazolone and IR treatment inhibited ATC cell growth [7]. Numerous SA-β-Gal–positive cells were markedly increased when anthrapyrazolone was combined with IR (Figure 14).

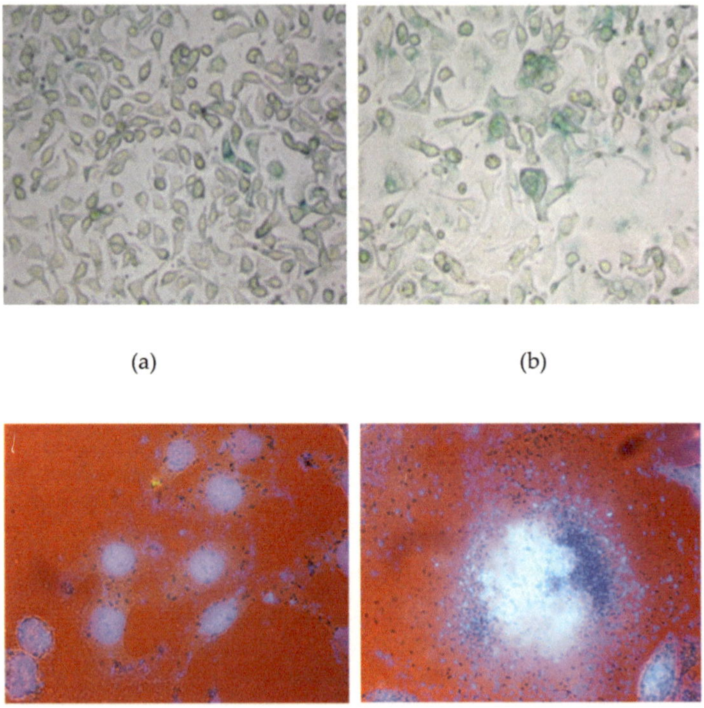

(a) (b)

(c) (d)

Figure 11. IR induces SLP associated with terminal growth arrest in human ATC cell lines: (a and c) non-irradiated; (b and d) in 120 hours after 10 Gy IR treatment; ATC cells exhibited typical features of SLP. Induction of SA-β-Gal activity (green) was mostly observed in large cells with increased granularity and flattened shape. SA-β-Gal staining method. (a) and (b) Bright-field microscopy, original magnification ×200. (c) and (d) Confocal fluorescent microscopy; original magnification ×400.

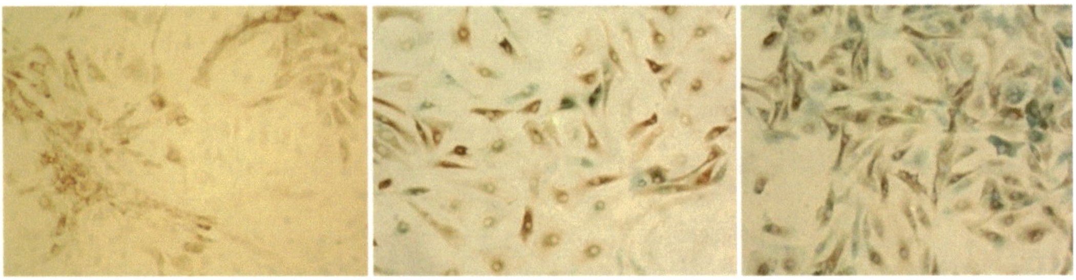

(a) (b) (c)

Figure 12. IR-induced SA-β-Gal activity in the primary culture of human thyroid follicular cells: (a) thyroglobulin-positive (brown) cells in primary culture, anti-thyroglobulin immunocytochemistry; (b) non-irradiated cells, double staining for SA-β-Gal and thyroglobulin; and (c) in 120 hours after 10 Gy IR treatment, double staining for SA-β-Gal and thyroglobulin. Original magnification ×200.

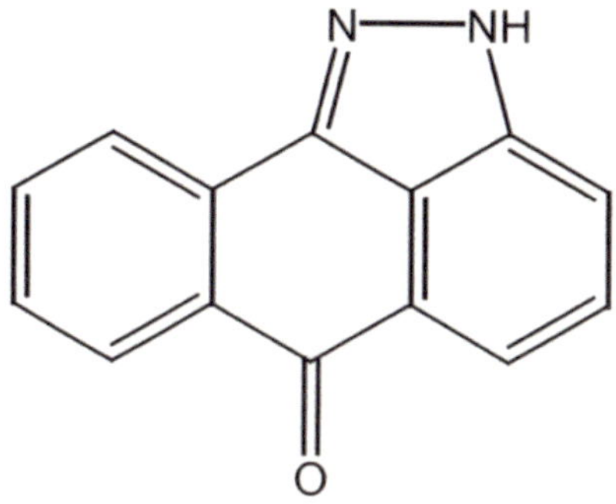

Figure 13. Chemical structure of anthrapyrazolone.

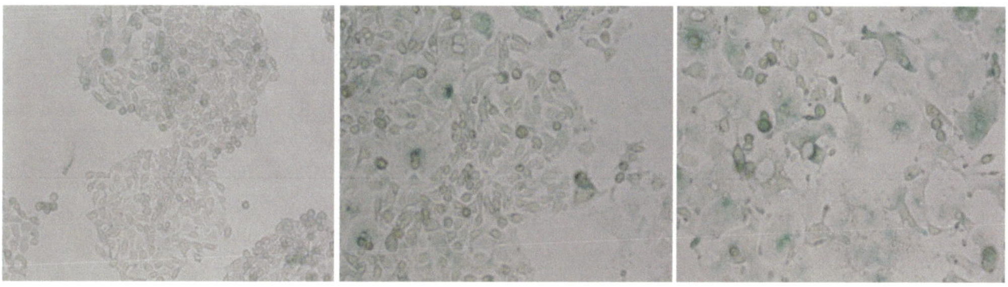

(a) (b) (c)

Figure 14. Anthrapyrazolone potentiates SLP in irradiated ATC cells: (a) non-radiated; (b) treatment with anthrapyrazolone; and (c) in 120 hours after 10 Gy IR treatment combined with anthrapyrazolone. SA-β-Gal staining method. Bright-field microscopy. Original magnification ×100.

It was observed a robust increase of tail moment (Figure 15), which represents DNA damage in alkaline single cell gel electrophoresis (Comet assay), in ATC cells treated with anthrapyrazolone plus IR compared to IR alone, suggesting that inhibition of JNK signaling pathway retarded DNA repair [7].

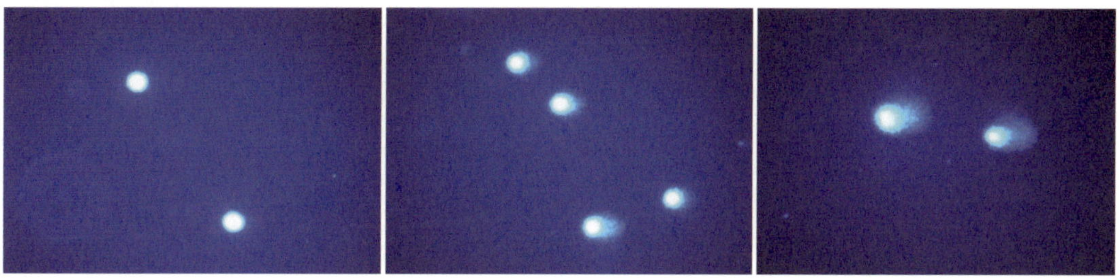

(a) (b) (c)

Figure 15. Anthrapyrazolone potentiates DNA damage in irradiated ATC cells: (a) non-radiated; (b) in 30 minutes after 10 Gy IR treatment; and (c) in 5 minutes after 10 Gy IR treatment combined with anthrapyrazolone. UV-fluorescent microscope.

In this study, DNA repair rates after 10 Gy exposure were analyzed by Comet assay to explore whether SLP induced by combination of anthrapyrazolone plus IR was associated with accumulation of DNA damage. In this method, individual cells with damaged DNA embedded in agarose gels are subjected to an electric field and generate a characteristic pattern of DNA distribution forming a tail that, after staining with fluorescence dye, can be analyzed by fluorescence microscopy. The extent and length of the comet's tail correlates with the severity of DNA damage [39].

Thus, one of the mechanisms that may contribute to the combination treatment effects is likely the delay of DNA repair evoked by JNK pathway inhibition. Treatment with anthrapyrazolone significantly delayed DNA rejoining after 10 Gy IR and increased the radiosensitivity of ATC cells.

7. Imatinib as a selective inhibitor of c-ABL tyrosine kinase activity

Imatinib (also known as STI571 or Gleevec®) is a tyrosine kinase inhibitor with selectivity toward BCR/ABL, c-ABL, platelet-derived growth factor receptor (PDGFR), and c-KIT (Figure 16) [40].

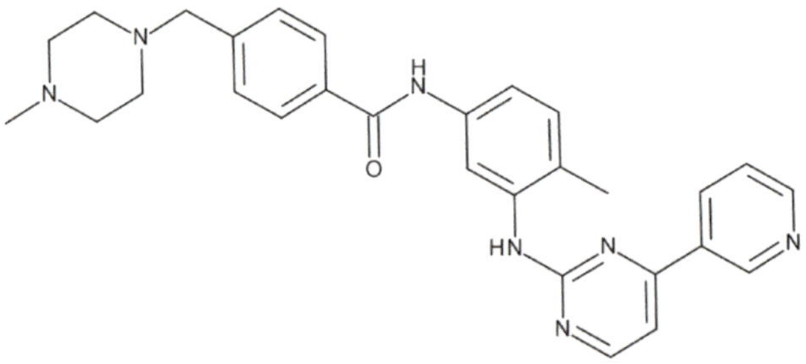

Figure 16. Chemical structure of imatinib.

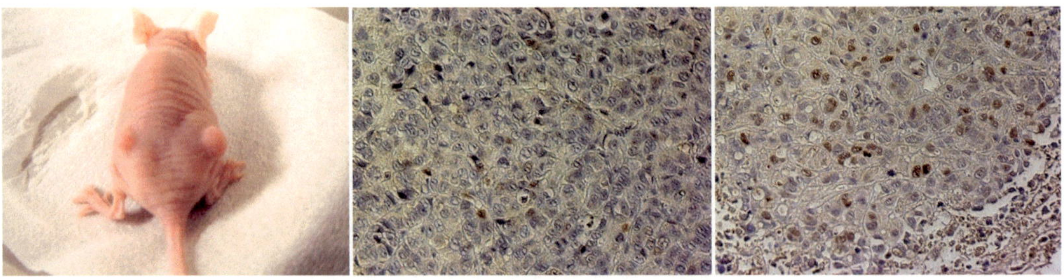

(a) (b) (c)

Figure 17. (a) ATC xenograft model (ATC cells were implanted s.c. into male athymic mice); (b) cell cycle inhibitor p21[cip1] expression in non-radiated mouse ATC cells xenograft; (c) imatinib 10 μM combined with single dose of 10 Gy IR in 120 hours after treatment. Imatinib suppressed *in vivo* growth of ATC cells implanted into nude mice. (b and c) immunohistochemistry, antibodies used were anti-p21[cip1]. Original magnification ×200.

Imatinib impedes the growth of ATC cell lines *in vitro* through selective inhibition of c-ABL tyrosine kinase activity [41]. *In vivo*, imatinib combined with IR promotes p21[cip1] expression in mice bearing ATC xenograft model (Figure 17).

It was demonstrated that imatinib-induced S- and G2–M cell cycle arrest, leading to cell growth inhibition (Figure 18) [41].

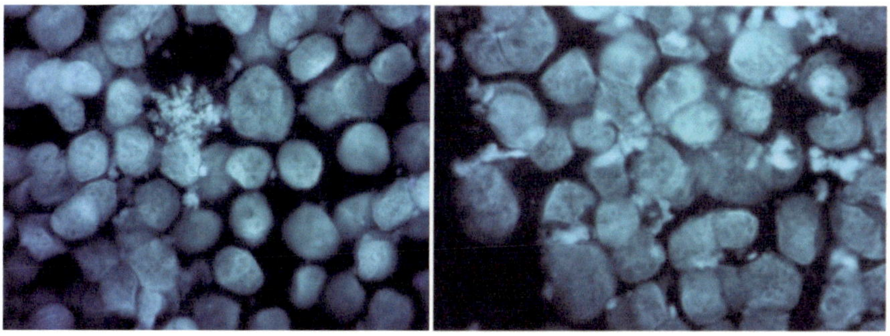

(a) (b)

Figure 18. To evaluate G2 arrest in ATC cells, changes in the percent mitotic cells should be determined: (a) in 120 hours after imatinib (10 μM) treatment and (b) in 120 hours after imatinib (10 μM) combined with single dose of 5 Gy IR treatment.

The anti-tumor effect of imatinib is potentiated in adjunctive therapy with IR, not only due to inhibition of proliferative cell growth with transient cell cycle arrest and apoptosis but also due to the terminal growth arrest associated with SLP (Figure 19) [41].

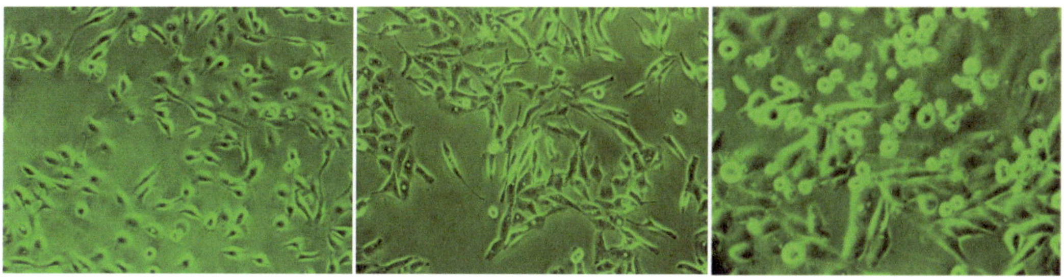

(a) (b) (c)

Figure 19. Phenotypic changes associated with SLP in ATC cells: (a) ATC cell line without treatment; (b) in 72 hours after imatinib (10 μM) treatment; (c) in 72 hours after imatinib (10 μM) treatment combined with single dose of 5 Gy IR. Enlarged and flattened morphology and increased granularity of ATC cells. Original magnification ×200.

8. Conclusion

Intracellular JNK and c-ABL signaling pathways are essential components of ATC cell proliferation and survival after radiation therapy. Hence, pharmacological inhibition of these pathways in combination with radiotherapy may be a potential treatment modality of ATC.

Author details

Dmitry Bulgin[1*] and Alexey Podcheko[2]

*Address all correspondence to: molmed1999@yahoo.com

1 Center for Regenerative Medicine "ME-DENT", Rovinj, Croatia

2 American University of Integrative Sciences, St. Maarten School of Medicine, Sint Maarten, Caribbean Netherlands

References

[1] Ain KB. Anaplastic thyroid carcinoma: behavior, biology, and therapeutic approaches. Thyroid 1998;8:715–726. DOI:10.1089/thy.1998.8.715

[2] Namba H, Hara T, Tukazaki T, *et al.* Radiation-induced G1 arrest is selectively mediated by the p53-WAF1/Cip1 pathway in human thyroid cells. Cancer Res. 1995;55:2075–2080.

[3] Yang T, Namba H, Hara T, *et al.* p53 induced by ionizing radiation mediates DNA end-jointing activity, but not apoptosis of thyroid cells. Oncogene 1997;14:1511–1519.

[4] Heron DE, Karimpour S, Grigsby PW. Anaplastic thyroid carcinoma: comparison of conventional radiotherapy and hyperfractionation chemoradiotherapy in two groups. Am J Clin Oncol. 2002;25:442–446.

[5] Harari PM, Huang SM. Modulation of molecular targets to enhance radiation. Clin Cancer Res. 2000;6:323–325.

[6] Bianco C, Bianco R, Tortora G, *et al.* Antitumor activity of combined treatment of human cancer cells with ionizing radiation and anti-epidermal growth factor receptor monoclonal antibody C225 plus type I protein kinase A antisense oligonucleotide. Clin Cancer Res. 2000;6:4343–4350.

[7] Bulgin D, Podtcheko A, Takakura S, *et al*. Selective pharmacologic inhibition of c-Jun NH2-terminal kinase radiosensitizes thyroid anaplastic cancer cell lines via induction of terminal growth arrest. Thyroid 2006;16:217–224. DOI:10.1089/thy.2006.16.217

[8] Verheij M. Clinical biomarkers and imaging for radiotherapy-induced cell death. Cancer Metastasis Rev. 2008;27:471–480. DOI:10.1007/s10555-008-9131-1

[9] Baskar R, Lee KA, Yeo R, Yeoh KW. Cancer and radiation therapy: current advances and future directions. Int J Med Sci. 2012;9:193–199. DOI:10.7150/ijms.3635

[10] Rogakou EP, Pilch DR, Orr AH, Ivanova VS, Bonner WM. DNA double-stranded breaks induce histone H2AX phosphorylation on serine 139. J Biol Chem. 1998;273:5858–5868. DOI:10.1074/jbc.273.10.5858

[11] Podhorecka M, Skladanowski A, Bozko P. H2AX phosphorylation: its role in DNA damage response and cancer therapy. J Nucl Acids. 2010;2010:920161. DOI: 10.4061/2010/920161

[12] Huang X, Halicka HD, Traganos F, Tanaka T, Kurose A, Darzynkiewicz Z. Cytometric assessment of DNA damage in relation to cell cycle phase and apoptosis. Cell Proliferat. 2005;38:223–243. DOI:10.1111/j.1365-2184.2005.00344.x

[13] Darzynkiewicz Z, Huang X, Okafuji M. Detection of DNA strand breaks by flow and laser scanning cytometry in studies of apoptosis and cell proliferation (DNA replication). Methods Mol Biol. 2006;314:81–93. DOI:10.1385/1-59259-973-7:081

[14] Eriksson D, Stigbrand T. Radiation-induced cell death mechanisms. Tumour Biol. 2010;31:363–372. DOI:10.1007/S13277-010-0042-8

[15] Hibi M, Lin A, Smeal T, Minden A, Karin M. Identification of an oncoprotein- and UV-responsive protein kinase that binds and potentiates the c-Jun activation domain. Genes Dev. 1993;7:2135–2148. DOI:10.1101/gad.7.11.2135

[16] Davis RJ. MAPKs: new JNK expands the group. Trends Biochem Sci. 1994;19:470–473.

[17] Prasad MV, Dermott JM, Heasley LE, *et al.* Activation of Jun kinase/stress-activated protein kinase by GTPase-deficient mutants of G alpha 12 and G alpha 13. J Biol Chem. 1995;270:18655–18659. DOI:10.1074/jbc.270.31.18655

[18] Westwick JK, Weitzel C, Minden A, *et al.* Tumor necrosis factor alpha stimulates AP-1 activity through prolonged activation of the c-Jun kinase. J Biol Chem. 1994;269:26396–26401.

[19] Cano E, Hazzalin CA, Mahadevan LC. Anisomycin-activated protein kinases p45 and p55 but not mitogen-activated protein kinases ERK-1 and -2 are implicated in the induction of c-fos and c-jun. Mol Cell Biol. 1994;14:7352–7362. DOI:10.1128/MCB.14.11.7352

[20] Watters D. Molecular mechanisms of ionizing radiation-induced apoptosis. Immunol Cell Biol. 1999;77:263–271. DOI:10.1046/J.1440-1711.1999.00824.X

[21] Kuwabara M, Takahashi K, Inanami O. Induction of apoptosis through the activation of SAPK/JNK followed by the expression of death receptor Fas in X-irradiated cells. J Radiat Res. 2003;44:203–209.

[22] Davis RJ. Signal transduction by the JNK group of MAP kinases. Cell 2000;103:239–252. DOI:10.1016/S0092-8674(00)00116-1

[23] Van Etten R.A. Cycling, stressed-out and nervous: cellular functions of c-ABL. Trends Cell Biol. 1999;9:179–186. DOI:10.1016/S0962-8924(99)01549-4

[24] Greuber EK, Smith-Pearson P, Wang J, Pendergast AM. Role of ABL family kinases in cancer: from leukaemia to solid tumours. Nat Rev Cancer. 2013;13:559–571. DOI: 10.1038/nrc3563

[25] Cheng L, Lloyd RV, Weaver AL, *et al.* The cell cycle inhibitors p21WAF1 and p27KIP1 are associated with survival in patients treated by salvage prostatectomy after radiation therapy. Clin Cancer Res. 2000;6:1896–1899.

[26] Yoshida K, Miki Y. Enabling death by the ABL tyrosine kinase: mechanisms for nuclear shuttling of c-ABL in response to DNA damage. Cell Cycle 2005;4:777–779.

[27] Shafman T, Khanna KK, Kedar P, *et al.* Interaction between ATM protein and c-ABL in response to DNA damage. Nature 1997;387:520–523. DOI:10.1038/387520a0

[28] Podtcheko A, Ohtsuru A, Namba H, *et al.* Inhibition of ABL tyrosine kinase potentiates radiation-induced terminal growth arrest in anaplastic thyroid cancer cells. Radiat Res. 2006;165:35–42.

[29] Yuan ZM, Huang Y, Whang Y, *et al.* Role for c-ABL tyrosine kinase in growth arrest response to DNA damage. Nature 1996;382:272–274. DOI:10.1038/382272a0

[30] Sionov RV, Moallem E, Berger M, *et al.* c-ABL neutralizes the inhibitory effect of Mdm2 on p53. J Biol Chem. 1999;274:8371–8374. DOI:10.1074/jbc.274.13.8371

[31] Ito T, Seyama T, Mizuno T, *et al.* Unique association of p53 mutations with undifferentiated but not with differentiated carcinomas of the thyroid gland. Cancer Res. 1992;52:1369–1371.

[32] Fagin JA, Matsuo K, Karmakar A, *et al.* High prevalence of mutations of the p53 gene in poorly differentiated human thyroid carcinomas. J Clin Invest. 1993;91:179–184. DOI:10.1172/JCI116168

[33] Namba H, Hara T, Tukazaki T, *et al.* Radiation-induced G1 arrest is selectively mediated by the p53-WAF1/Cip1 pathway in human thyroid cells. Cancer Res. 1995;55:2075–2080.

[34] Whang YE, Tran C, Henderson C, *et al.* c-ABL is required for development and optimal cell proliferation in the context of p53 deficiency. Proc Natl Acad Sci USA. 2000;97:5486–5491.

[35] Schmitt CA. Cellular senescence and cancer treatment. Biochim Biophys Acta. 2007;1775:5–20. DOI:10.1016/j.bbcan.2006.08.005

[36] Podtcheko A, Namba H, Saenko V, *et al.* Radiation-induced senescence-like terminal growth arrest in thyroid cells. Thyroid 2005;15:306–313. DOI:10.1089/thy.2005.15.306

[37] Bennett BL, Sasaki DT, Murray BW, *et al.* SP600125, an anthrapyrazolone inhibitor of Jun N-terminal kinase. Proc Natl Acad Sci USA. 2001;98:13681–13686. DOI:10.1073/pnas.251194298

[38] Gururajan M, Chui R, Karuppannan AK, *et al.* c-Jun N-terminal kinase (JNK) is required for survival and proliferation of B-lymphoma cells. Blood 2005;106:1382–1391. DOI:10.1182/blood-2004-10-3819

[39] Ostling O, Johanson KJ. Microelectrophoretic study of radiation-induced DNA damages in individual mammalian cells. Biochem Biophys Res Commun. 1984;123:291–298. DOI:10.1016/0006-291X(84)90411-X

[40] Krystal GW, Honsawek S, Litz J, Buchdunger E. The selective tyrosine kinase inhibitor STI571 inhibits small cell lung cancer growth. Clin Cancer Res. 2000;6:3319–3326.

[41] Podtcheko A, Ohtsuru A, Tsuda S, *et al.* The selective tyrosine kinase inhibitor, STI571, inhibits growth of anaplastic thyroid cancer cells. J Clin Endocrinol Metab. 2003;88:1889–1896. DOI:10.1210/jc.2002-021230

Chapter 7

Modern Technologies for Timely Detection and Differential Diagnosis of Gastric Cancer

Vladimir Levkin, Nina Gagarina, Sergey Kharnas, Gaziyav Musaev, Artem Shiryaev and Dmitry Bulgin

Additional information is available at the end of the chapter

http://dx.doi.org/10.5772/62540

Abstract

The diagnostic potentialities of laser spectro- and videofluorescence endoscopy, complex transabdominal US examination, dynamic multihelical computed tomography (MHCT) with the possibility of constructing multiplanar reformations, and virtual gastroscopy were studied with a view to diagnosing gastric cancer (GC). It was established that laser spectral fluorescence with the drug Alasens (5-aminolevulinic acid) is a highly revealing method for diagnosis and differential diagnosis of GC. The sensitivity of the method is 96%, and its specificity is 78%. Well-defined videofluorescence was noted in 91.3% of patients with GC. The possibility of detecting cancer with complex trans-ultrasonography in the pyloroantral division and in the lower third of the body of the stomach constitutes 95.6% attaining absolute values in T3 and T4. Dynamic MHCT allows 97% detection of GC attaining absolute values, beginning with T2 invasion depth; tumor localization is irrelevant. Comparative visual assessment of the quality of a virtual image and conventional video esophagogastroduodenoscopy (EGDS) was made. The study demonstrated a sufficiently high level of virtual images whose quality was not inferior to that of conventional images in intraluminal tumor growth. The indications for the application of this technique require further specification.

Keywords: Gastric cancer, 5-aminolevulinic acid (Alasens), laser spectro- and videofluorescence, complex transabdominal US examination, dynamic multihelical-computed tomography, virtual endoscopy

1. Introduction

Despite the fact that during the previous decades the incidence of gastric cancer (GC) has been tending to decrease in many countries of the world, this disease continues to occupy a leading place in the structure of oncological diseases and is one of the commonest causes of death from malignant neoplasms [1]. It is common knowledge that the success of treatment of patients with GC primarily depends on the timely diagnosis (tumor detection or primary diagnosis).

The main methods that enable us to detect gastric tumor and to verify the diagnosis are esophagogastroduodenoscopy with biopsy and roentgenologic examination of the upper gastrointestinal tract using the double contrast technique. The advantages of these methods are known and indisputable. At the same time, their shortcomings are also well known, namely the difficulty in detecting early forms of cancer as well as tumors with the endophytic submucosal character of growth. A relatively high number of both false-negative and false-positive results necessitates repeat endoscopic examinations and biopsies [2].

At present, laser fluorescence spectroscopy is one of the promising methods for the early diagnosis of malignant tumors, including GC [3, 4]. This method allows us to enhance the efficacy of the standard endoscopic examination in cancer and proved so informative that it is referred to as 'optic biopsy.' We distinguish autofluorescence, i.e., fluorescence of endogenic porphyrins whose concentration in the tumor cells is higher than in normal cells, and secondary fluorescence, i.e., the fluorescence of special exogenous photosensitizers, which are tropic to tumor cells. Neither method is free from typical disadvantages: photosensitizers are accumulated not only in the tumor but also in the skin and visible mucous membranes where they are retained for a long time and cause photodermatitis if the light regimen is compromised. The main disadvantages of autofluorescence monitoring are a low contrast ratio and the necessity of high-precision costly equipment.

Laser fluorescence spectroscopy has offered new possibilities with the development of 5-aminolevulinic acid (5-ALA), which induces the synthesis and accumulation of photoactive protoporphyrin IX in tumor cells. This results in intense fluorescence, which can be registered not only with spectroanalyzers but also with special highly sensitive fluorescent endoscopes, which opens up new horizons for clinical practice.

With the appearance of new radiodiagnostic technologies and the perfection of the already available [such as ultrasonography, endo-ultrasonography, computed tomography (CT), magnetic resonance imaging, and positron emission tomography] techniques, their possibilities in modern diagnostics of GC are actively being assessed [5–7]. In particular, numerous investigations demonstrated the potentialities of a complex transabdominal US examination with water loading as a method for primary diagnosis of GC [5].

Computed tomography is conventionally considered to be a method for secondary diagnosis of GC and, above all, detection of remote metastases. However, the studies conducted recently give evidence of the fact that the results of multihelical computed tomography (MHCT) are on a par with those of the X-ray and endoscopic methods in detecting GC [8]. Moreover, this method allows, after preliminarily insufflating the stomach, the performance of the so-called virtual gastroscopy. Thus, dynamic MHCT additionally allows a wider field of view of the organ in the modes of constructing multiplanar reformations and virtual endoscopy and, in contrast to conventional videoendoscopy, is characterized by the absence of blind zones [7, 9]. The drawbacks of the method are as follows: the construction of multiplanar and virtual images is time-consuming; the absence of delicate shades of color at the boundary of lesion; the impossibility to perform biopsy; and radiation exposure [7, 9]. Most of the works devoted to primary diagnostics of GC with MHCT are mainly of pilot character.

The aim of this study is to look into the diagnostic possibilities of laser spectro- and video-fluorescent endoscopy, complex trans-US examination, MHCT with the possibility of constructing multiplanar reformations, and virtual gastroscopy in the primary diagnosis of GC.

2. Materials and methods

The studies were conducted in the Burdenko Surgical Clinic of the Sechenov First Moscow State Medical University from 2003 to 2010.

The results of laser spectral fluorescence diagnostics (FD) were analyzed in 62 patients with malignant (37, 59.7%) and benign (35, 40.3%) diseases. Videofluorescence was observed in 25 patients (23 with GC and 2 with benign diseases). The study was conducted using 5-ALA–based Alasens (GNTs NIOPIK, Research Institute of Organic Semi-Products and Dyes), which was preliminarily dissolved in 200 mL of water (10–20 mg/kg of body mass) and ingested per os 1.5–2 h before the study. A LESA-01 spectroanalyzer (Biospek and the Institute of Optic Physics, Russian Academy of Sciences, Russia) was used for monitoring fluorescence. To pinpoint videofluorescence (Figure 2), a special attachment for the standard endoscope consisting of a high-sensitivity camera (0.003 lx) and a system of light filters and a photodiode laser with a wavelength of 630 nm and a power of 1.5 W were used.

Eighty-seven patients with GC underwent complex trans-US examination. The study was conducted using SIQUOIA apparatuses (ACUSON, the United States) operating in the real-time mode and furnished with a convex transducer with a frequency of 2.5–3.5 MHz and a linear probe with a frequency of 7.0–11.0 MHz. A two-stage method with the water test proposed by Worlicek et al. (1989) was used when ultrasonography was performed [9].

Ninety patients with verified GC and 10 patients with suspected GC were subjected to dynamic MHCT. The study was conducted using a Toshiba 320-slice tomograph with 16-cm detector that allowed three-dimensional (3D) dynamic scanning with visualization of the whole stomach in the dynamic mode without table feed. The native sequence was then performed, a 16-cm examination zone along the Z-axis (embracing the whole stomach) was chosen, and the abdominal cavity and the small pelvis were scanned. The subsequent procedure included the construction of multiplanar reformations and dynamic video files. When virtual gastroscopy was constructed (16 patients), the stomachs were preliminarily insufflated through a probe or by using a special effervescent mixture consisting of citric acid and sodium bicarbonate (4.0–6.0 g).

To objectively evaluate the information content of the methods used for diagnosing GC and assessing its extent of spread, the diagnostic results were compared with the intraoperative and histological findings. The international TNM classification (UICC 2002) was used for staging GC.

The clinical data were analyzed with the standard methods for statistical processing using Microsoft Excel, SPSS 14.0, and MedCalc 5.0.

3. Results

3.1. Laser spectral and videofluorescent diagnostics of gastric cancer

Only 18 patients were diagnosed as having GC prior to the performance of FD. Later, this diagnosis was verified by both the fluorescence intensity data (PRIX, the contrast ratio 2.1–18.6) and histological findings.

Of 31 patients with the preliminary diagnosis of gastric ulcer, FD performance revealed a high-fluorescence intensity (the contrast ratio 2.1–9.6) at the edges of ulceration in 12 patients (Figure 1).

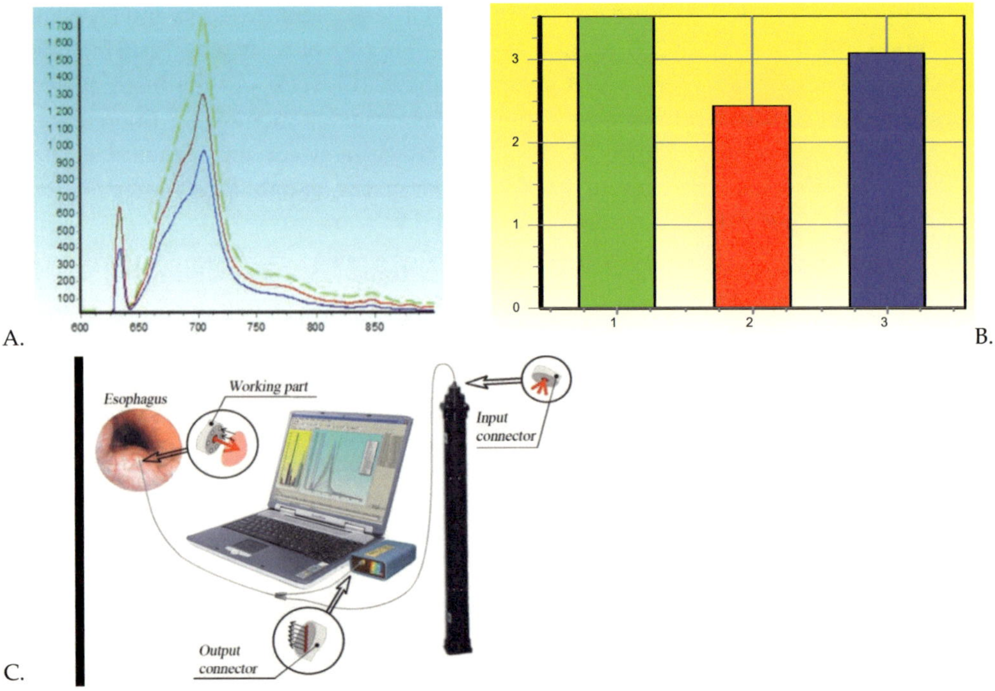

Figure 1. (A) Spectrogram and (B) histogram in gastric cancer and (C) the scheme and the principle of operation of LESA-01.

Target biopsy of the mucous membrane was performed at these points; histological examination of the biopsy material confirmed the diagnosis of GC. In the remaining 14 patients, the FD data (the contrast ratio 0.7–0.8) coincided with the histological findings; the diagnosis of gastric ulcer was verified.

Esophagogastroduodenoscopy revealed atypical regions of the mucosa suggestive of cancer in five patients. High-intensity fluorescence of ALA-induced PRIX (the contrast ratio 2.1–8.0) was observed in four patients when FD was carried out. Target biopsy of the mucous membrane of the stomach was performed, and the diagnosis of GC was made. Likewise, a patient with a gastric polyp (the contrast ratio 3.3) was diagnosed as having carcinoma in situ based on the results of histological examination.

In four patients, the preliminary diagnosis of GC was rejected after spectroscopy, which was verified by the data of the subsequent morphological examination.

High-intensity fluorescence of ALA-induced PRIX was detected at 1–2 points of the region studied in five observations. As evidenced by the results of histological examination, a markedly pronounced inflammatory reaction was revealed in four of five of these patients. Numerous authors [3] report that inflammation may be associated with increased generation of ALA-induced PPIX.

Taking into account the foregoing, these patients can be included in the risk group but not assigned to those with false-positive results. These patients require preventive endoscopic examinations at least once a year.

In one observation, during FD the contrast ratio constituted 1.1; however, morphological examination revealed highly differentiated adenocarcinoma. This result can be attributed to false-negative ones.

On the whole, the contrast ratio constituted 4.55 ± 0.2 across the GC group (from 3.83 ± 0.6 in carcinoma in situ to 6.13 ± 0.2 in stage IV). In patients with gastric ulcer, the contrast ratio was 1.08 ± 0.7. The difference between the contrast ratio values in malignant and benign diseases is statistically significant ($p \leq 0.05$). The sensitivity of the diagnostic method with the study of Alasens-induced fluorescence was 96%, and its specificity was 78%.

3.2. Videofluorescence study

When performing endoscopic examination of the fluorescent images of the stomach, distinct fluorescence of the tumor in 21 (91.3%) of 23 patients with GC was noted (Figure 2).

In two patients, the diagnosis of GC was excluded during complex examination and, accordingly, videofluorescence was absent (no false-negative results were noted). In addition, the foci of severe dysplasia and malignancy were seen to be fluorescing, which was later confirmed by the results of analysis of both the fluorescence spectra and the biopsy findings.

3.3. Complex trans-ultrasonography in the primary diagnosis of GC

To assess the possibilities of complex transabdominal US examination as a potential screening method in detecting GC, we examined patients with different stages and different localization of the neoplastic process.

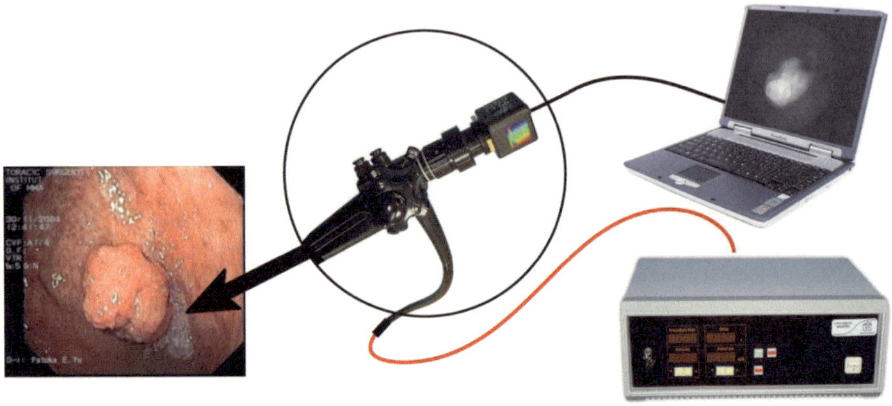

A.

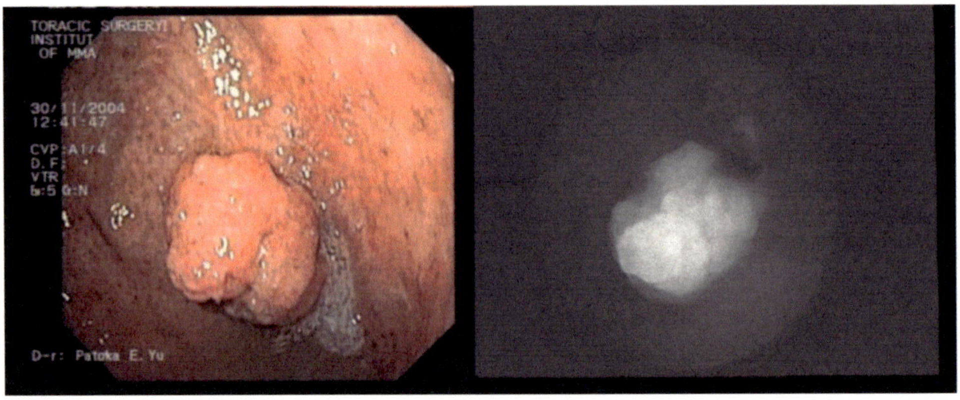

B.

Figure 2. (A) Prototype of the videofluorescence unit and (B) Malignant gastric polyp (videoendoscopy and video-fluorescence).

3.3.1. T1 invasion depth

To reveal disease at this stage of development of the pathological process is a difficult task due to a small short local extension and a low depth of the tumor lesion (Figure 3).

According to the postoperative histological findings, 28 patients had T2 invasion depth; the performance of ultrasonography was successful in detecting the tumor in 20 patients (in 8 patients using the standard technique; in 12 patients, US + ingestion of water). In six observations, the tumor was localized in the regions inaccessible to US examination: the cardia and the upper third of the stomach body; in two observations, in the pyloroantral zone and the lower third of the body at the lesser curvature.

In two observations, ultrasonography was the first diagnostic procedure that enabled us to suspect early antral cancer in the form of local thickening of the gastric wall with 1.5-cm

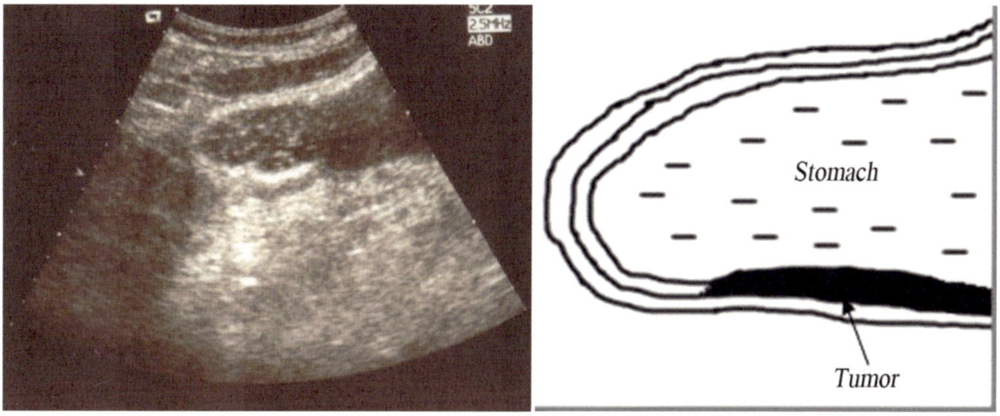

A. B.

Figure 3. (A) Echogram and (B) the scheme of the infiltrative lesion of the gastric wall. T1 invasion depth.

extension, which was subsequently verified by the esophagogastroduodenoscopy (EGDS) + biopsy and X-ray findings.

Thus, complex US examination was instrumental in detecting a tumor at T1 invasion depth in 72% of observations, and when the tumor was localized in the pyloroantral division of the stomach and in the lower third of the organ, this level increased to 90%. The sensitivity and specificity of this technique in measuring the T1 invasion depth constituted 42.9% and 91.8%, respectively.

3.3.2. T2 invasion depth

According to the histological findings, T2 invasion depth was noted in 19 patients; complex ultrasonography revealed a tumor in 18 patients. In one patient, the tumor was localized in the cardiac region and in the upper third of the stomach body, i.e., the regions inaccessible to US examination. At the first stage of complex US examination, a tumor was detected in 16 patients and in two more patients at the second stage with the water test. However, in numerous cases, it was not simple to reveal a tumor with category T2 invasion depth. This was only possible when the organ was thoroughly and meticulously examined.

Thus, the detection rate for T2 invasion depth lesions was 95% if the tumor was localized in the pyloric and antral divisions of the stomach or involved in its body. The sensitivity and specificity in determining T2 invasion depth constituted 63.2% and 81%, respectively.

3.3.3. T3 invasion depth

According to the histological findings, T3 invasion depth was noted in 16 patients. In all observations, except one (a tumor invading the upper third and the cardiac division of the stomach with a low degree of extension), we succeeded in detecting the tumor easily enough resorting to both techniques: the standard ultrasonography and US supplemented with water loading. At this depth of lesion, it was the classical 'hollow organ' symptom that was most commonly observed in the US image. At this pathological stage, we visualized not only considerable thickening of the stomach wall but also a large extent of spread of the tumor along the longitudinal axis of the organ involving several anatomical regions. All this facilitated the task of tumor detection.

Thus, ultrasound examination supplemented with the water test did not increase the information content in terms of tumor detection at this stage of the disease but allowed us to evaluate more thoroughly the extent of infiltration, to determine the depth of involvement by the tumor, and to improve visualization of the organs of the retroperitoneal space.

Complex transabdominal US examination enabled us to reveal the tumor in 94% of cases in T3 invasion depth. If the localization site was the pylorus, antrum, and body of the stomach, the detection rate was 100%. The sensitivity and specificity in relation to measuring the invasion depth were 75% and 83.6%, respectively.

3.3.4. T4 invasion depth

As judged by the results of the histological examination of biopsy material, T4 invasion depth was noted in 14 patients. In all the observations of patients with category T4 malignant lesions, the tumor was revealed easily as the 'hollow organ' symptom due to a large extent of spread using both techniques: the standard ultrasonography and US with water loading.

In our study, invasion of the adjacent organs, the great vessels, and fatty tissue by the tumor was suspected during ultrasonic examination in four patients, which was later confirmed intraoperatively using the same procedure and by revision of the organs of the abdominal cavity.

Thus, the possibility of detecting tumor lesions of the stomach with T4 invasion depth was absolute. As far as the sensitivity and specificity of the method are concerned, they are 85.7% and 93.7%, respectively.

3.4. Dynamic MHCT in the diagnostics of gastric cancer

Until recently, CT was regarded as a technique for secondary diagnosis of GC. As dynamic MHCT is a more informative diagnostic method, we studied the possibilities of primary diagnostics of GC, including the so-called virtual endoscopy.

3.4.1. T1 invasion depth

Based on the data of postoperative histological examination, T1 invasion depth was diagnosed in nine patients. We succeeded in detecting the tumor in seven of nine observations (78%). In all the cases, T1 invasion depth was characterized by the non-uniform contrast of the mucous–submucous layer and peristaltic disorder, even if the wall thickening was insignificant. In two observations of early GC (carcinoma in situ), we failed to reveal the tumor.

Thus, the sensitivity of MHCT in revealing T1 invasion depth constituted 22%; its specificity is 100%; the positive predictive value (PPV) is 100%; and the negative predictive value (NPV) is 93%.

3.4.2. *T2 invasion depth*

According to the histological findings, T2 invasion depth was determined in 13 patients. We succeeded in detecting the tumor in all the cases, irrespective of the localization of the neoplastic process in the stomach.

The most characteristic CT symptom at T2 invasion depth, as at T1 invasion depth, is limited thickening of the gastric wall (13.6 ± 5.4 mm) with increased accumulation of the contrast medium and with impaired peristalsis in this division without the involvement of perigastric fatty tissue.

The sensitivity of MHCT in measuring T2 invasion depth constituted 69%; its specificity is 92%; PPV is 57%; and NPV is 95%.

3.4.3. *T3 invasion depth*

According to the results of histological examination, the T3 invasion depth group included 24 patients. With T3 invasion depth, marked (19.0 ± 8.4 mm) thickening of the stomach wall, irregularity of the external outline with reticular, and linear thickening of the surrounding fatty tissue are noted.

The accumulation of contrast medium by the tumor was of different character and depended, to a larger degree, on its histological variant. It was not difficult to reveal the tumor lesion at this stage of the process due to the extent of spread when compared to stage T2, not to mention T1. Moreover, at this stage of the disease, not only the stomach wall is significantly thickened, but also the tumor is more extended involving several anatomical regions of the stomach, which was especially well seen when multiplanar images were constructed.

The sensitivity of MHCT in revealing T3 invasion depth constituted 80%; its specificity is 85%; PPV is 71%; and NPV is 91%.

3.4.4. *T4 invasion depth*

It should be noted that the T4 invasion depth is associated with the most significant lesion of the organ in terms of depth and the extent of spread. In all our observations (36 patients), it was not difficult to reveal the tumor as with T3 malignant lesions. The CT picture of T4 invasion depth, as visualized with dynamic MHCT, was characterized by marked thickening of the stomach walls (21.3 ± 7.1 mm) with their indistinct outline, infiltration of the adjacent fatty tissue, the absence of the boundary between the gastric wall and the adjacent organs, and invasion of the surrounding organs by the tumor (Figure 4).

The detection of the tumor involving the adjacent organs and tissues was a significant criterion confirming the presence of this stage of disease. Thus, according to the data of our study, when

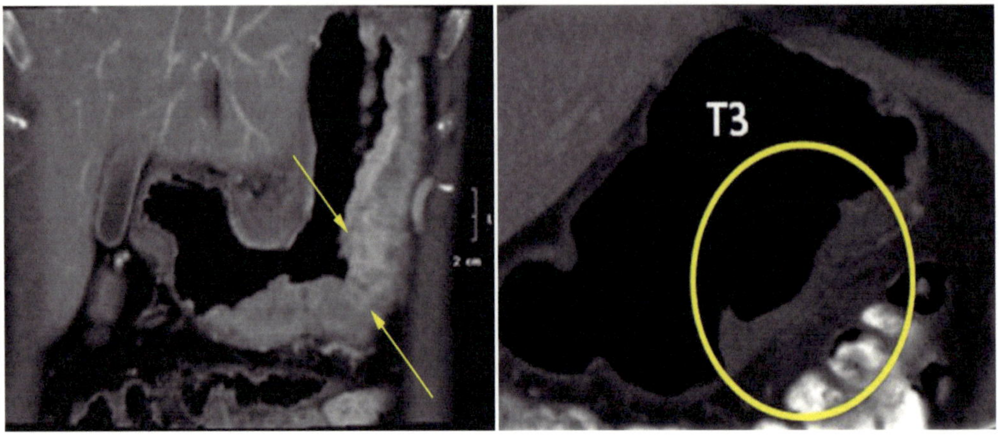

Figure 4. Dynamic MHCT, gastric cancer, subtotal lesion, T3–T4 invasion depth, multiplanar reformations.

MHCT was performed, we suspected invasion of the adjacent organs and the great vessels by the tumor in 18 patients, which was subsequently verified with intraoperative ultrasonographic examination and by revision of the organs of the abdominal cavity.

The sensitivity of MHCT in detecting T4 invasion depth was 83%; its specificity is 95%; PPV is 91%; and NPV is 91%.

On the whole, the sensitivity of MHCT in detecting GC constituted 97%; its specificity is 100%; PPV is 100%; and NPV is 77%.

3.5. Virtual endoscopy

Some authors consider virtual endoscopy as a potentially screening method of diagnostics and differential diagnostics of GC. In this connection, we evaluated the diagnostic possibilities of the method and the quality of the image obtained in the process of simulation.

3.5.1. Gastric leiomyoma

Based on the EGDS and X-ray data, two patients had intraluminal tumor growth; in one female patient, the tumor was localized outside the stomach only insignificantly bulging into the lumen of the organ. In all the cases, a virtual image obtained as a result of CT simulation was characterized by a high quality maximally approximating to the image obtained during videoendoscopy. The study enabled us to specify the localization of the tumor, and the planar slices demonstrated the tumor site relative to the stomach wall (intraparietal localization with prolapse into the lumen or extragastral). These data allowed us to preliminarily choose and plan the optimal treatment modality (wedge resection of the stomach was performed in all patients).

When a virtual image is constructed in patients with GC, it is worth pointing out the following. In the cases when exophytic tumor growth (Type 1, according to Bormann's classification) was

http://dx.doi.org/10.5772/62540

noted (three observations; Figure 5), the greatest similarity between a virtual and video image was obtained (irrespective of localization of the tumor in the stomach).

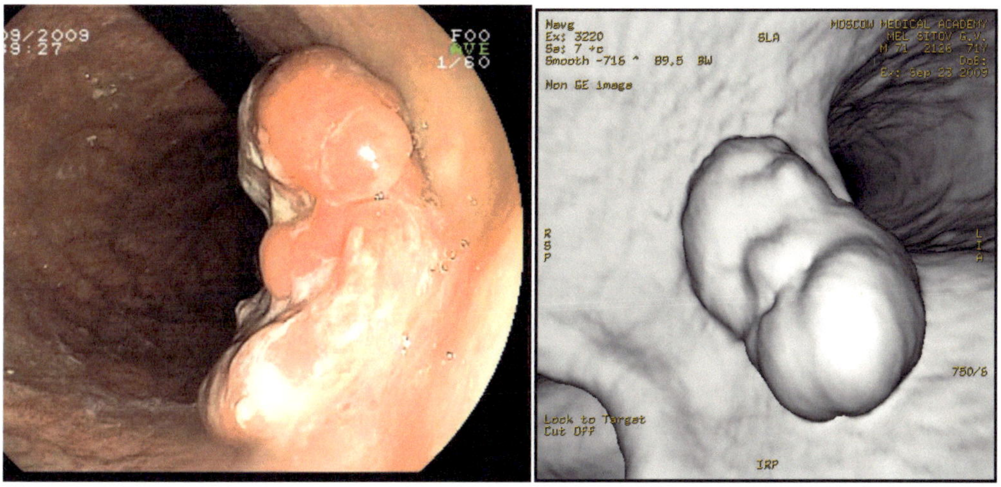

Figure 5. Video EGDS. The virtual endoscopy.

The high quality of virtual images was also noted in the infiltrative and mixed character of growth, when the tumor was localized in the body of the stomach (five patients). In infiltrative tumor growth with the phenomena of antral stenosis, the presence of fluid (primarily, its amount) in the organ lumen affected the quality of the image, which resulted in the appearance of artifacts in the simulation process (in two of five patients). Note that the mucous membrane in the region of lesion and nearby was characterized by excessive serration, although the circular narrowing of the antral division of the stomach characteristic of such a lesion was also well visualized as in videoendoscopy. The planar slices specified the depth of tumor invasion and the status of regional lymphatic vessels and allowed the detection of remote metastases. Unfortunately, the video sequences obtained during the study were characterized by the monotonousness of color images and did not allow us to pinpoint the areas of necrosis and disintegration, hemorrhage of the tumor surface, as well as perineoplastic and inflammatory mucosal changes. The high level (100%) of detection of a tumor lesion of the organ during virtual simulation in our study is determined by the vast extent of the lesion (large-sized leiomyomas and extended stage II–IV GC) and a good level of inflation of the organ.

4. Discussion

Despite rapid development of medical technologies, it is difficult to differentiate between benign and malignant tumors of the stomach. In this connection, the development of new and the perfection of available technologies is an important task. One of the most promising methods for increasing the resolving capacity of endoscopic examination is laser spectro- and videofluorescence. The procedure of endoscopic fluorescent diagnostics only insignificantly lengthens the EGDS performance time (in contrast to chromoendoscopy), and the conclusion as to the character of a pathological process can be formulated immediately in the process of gastroscopy performance. The equipment complex used now for FD is compact (portable) and mobile enough, which allows it to be delivered to the endoscopy room. No additional time for assembling the complex and preparing it for operation under the endoscopy room conditions is required. The rapid elimination of Alasens from the body decreases the likelihood of the development of toxic and photic reactions and makes it a drug of choice for fluorescent diagnostics. All the above mentioned allows us to recommend laser spectral FD combined with the study of Alasens-induced PPIX, and videofluorescence in the future, to use in the clinical setting as an express method of diagnosis, including the early diagnosis, of malignant gastric tumors.

This study showed that complex transabdominal ultrasonography is a highly informative method of diagnosis of GC. The possibility of detecting GC localized in the pyloroantral division and in the lower third of the stomach body during trans-US performance approaches the absolute values (97.4%). At the same time, in isolated lesions of the cardia and the upper third of the stomach body, we failed to reveal the tumor in any of the 10 patients studied. On the whole, the success rate of revealing GC at all tumor sites using complex trans-US examination constituted 87.0%. The high level of detection of the neoplastic process in the stomach in our study can be explained by the fact that we knew exactly where the process was localized in most patients (based on the EGDS and X-ray findings) and targeted at the zone concerned. However, this does not decrease the possibilities of the method but, on the contrary, testifies to its high diagnostic potential. In addition to the changes revealed for the first time in the stomach (in two patients with early cancer), the 'hollow organ' symptom was detected in numerous patients at the outpatient step followed by purpose-oriented examination and verification of the diagnosis with the subsequent referral to the clinic for operative treatment. Our experience shows that routine ultrasonography of the organs of the abdominal cavity should not be confined to the examination of the parenchymatous organs only. What is necessary is target visualization in the region of hollow organs (in particular, the stomach), especially in patients with the phenomena of abdominal discomfort. True, ultrasonography is actually the first and sometimes the only diagnostic procedure for most of such patients.

The studies conducted recently emphasized low diagnostic possibilities of conventional CT investigation in detecting GC, especially at stage T1 when the attempts to reveal any changes in the stomach wall were unsuccessful. On the whole, the accuracy of detecting the depth of invasion in more prevalent forms was not satisfactory either (no more than 65%) [10]. The main limiting factors were artifacts from peristaltic movements of the stomach wall, which did not allow us to assess its condition on standard examination. However, at present, the appearance of dynamic 3D MHCT capable of assessing the stomach wall in all the divisions in the four-dimensional mode has significantly increased the diagnostic possibilities of this technique.

In our study, dynamic 3D CT proved to be a highly revealing technique for GC (sensitivity 97%). Such high values were primarily achieved by virtue of the possibility of evaluating peristaltic disorders of the stomach, which was afforded by this CT technique, in contrast to the standard method relying on measuring only the thickness of the stomach wall. Dynamic MHCT enabled us to reveal seven of nine (85%) cases of early GC owing to the characteristic contrast between the mucous and submucous layers and peristaltic disorders without the stomach wall thickening. But it is fair to say that, at present, MHCT is inferior to the conventional endoscopic examination in revealing early GC.

The progress in computer technology led to the fact that virtual simulation is finding an ever wider application in different fields of surgery and oncology [6]. Our study demonstrated the possibilities of such simulation as applied to the construction of virtual gastroscopy. A high-quality virtual image not inferior to that acquired with conventional videoendoscopy was obtained in the case of intraluminal character of neoplastic growth [7, 9]. As it follows from the literature data, virtual endoscopy is not surpassed by conventional endoscopy in terms of its diagnostic possibilities of tumor detection and is more informative than planar slices, especially when the invasion depth is small (T2 and especially T1). Nevertheless, it is fair to say that now virtual endoscopy cannot be considered a real alternative to conventional videoendoscopy as a method of primary diagnostics of GC. At present, the possibilities of the wide application of the complex of CT techniques for differential diagnosis of benign and malignant ulcers with negative results of biopsy are also doubtful, although the first reports are highly encouraging [11]. In our opinion, the use of endo-ultrasonography and laser fluorescence spectroscopy (the so-called optic biopsy) is more justified for these purposes. Virtual simulation extends the possibilities of the method and allows for a more accurate choice of the target zone for a thorough study of the stomach wall with a view to specifying the depth of malignant invasion. However, the rapid progress of computer technology and software will possibly allow us to consider the complex of CT studies, including those in the virtual endoscopy mode, a screening technique in the countries with a high morbidity rate [7, 9]. At present, MHCT has found wide application in various diseases of the organs of the abdominal cavity, retroperitoneal space, and vertebral column. Therefore, we think that the use of such a method for an additional examination of the stomach in the group at higher risk not only for cancer but also for CT study of the organs of the abdominal cavity for other diseases with a view to detecting changes seems to be interesting and promising.

5. Conclusion

Fluorescent diagnostics with the study of Alasens-induced protoporphyrin IX is a highly efficacious, simple, and safe method for diagnosing GC. It can be used as a standard step of endoscopic examination in diagnostically complicated cases. The sensitivity of the method is 96%; its specificity is 98%.

The method for detecting videofluorescence with Alasens is a promising screening technique in patients with GC and in precancerous states.

Trans-ultrasonography is a potentially screening method in distal localization of GC. The possibility of detecting GC localized in the pyloroantral division and in the lower third of the body of the stomach using complex trans-ultrasonography was 95.6% attaining the absolute values in the T3 and T4 groups.

Dynamic MHCT is a highly informative method for cancer detection. The possibility of revealing cancer did not depend on the tumor localization and constituted 97% in the group of patients attaining absolute values, beginning with T2 invasion depth.

Indications for use of virtual endoscopy, one of the MHCT modes, as a method for the primary diagnosis of GC and for screening the disease require further study and specification.

Modern ultrasound and CT technologies allow us not only to stage GC but also to carry out primary diagnostics. However, the technical complexity and the high cost of CT, and the impossibility that cancer of the proximal division of the stomach will be detected ultrasonographically do not allow us to regard them as full-fledged screening techniques. Laser spectroscopy is indicated only in diagnostically difficult cases, and videofluorescent diagnostics requires higher performance, after which it may rightly be considered a recognized screening method.

Author details

Vladimir Levkin[1*], Nina Gagarina[1], Sergey Kharnas[1], Gaziyav Musaev[1], Artem Shiryaev[1] and Dmitry Bulgin[2]

*Address all correspondence to: doctor-levkin@mail.ru

1 Sechenov First Moscow State Medical University, Moscow, Russia

2 Center for Regenerative Medicine "ME-DENT", Rovinj, Croatia

References

[1] Davydov MI & Aksel EM. The incidence of malignant tumors and mortality caused by them in Commonwealth of Independent States in 2005. *Vestn Ross Akad Med Nauk,* 2007,11:45–49.

[2] Portnoi LM. Modern X-ray diagnostics in gastroenterology and gastroenterooncology. Moscow, Vidar-M, 2003.

[3] Polsachev VI. Preoperative fluorescent diagnostics of the prevalence of gastric cancer. *Vestn Khirurg,* 1989,12:17–19.

[4] Polsachev VI. Fluorescent method in the differential diagnosis of benign and malignant diseases of the stomach. *Vestn Khirurg,* 1992,1:95–97.

[5] Gorovaya NS. Role of complex US examination in the surgical treatment of gastric cancer patients. Cand. Sci. Dissertation (Med.), Moscow, 2009.

[6] Fedorov VD, Karamazovskii GG, Guzeeva EB & Tsvirkun VV. CT-based virtual surgical simulation. Moscow, Vidar-M, 2003.

[7] Kim JH, Eun HW, Choi JH, Hong SS, Kang W & Auh YH. Diagnostic performance of virtual gastroscopy using MDCT in early gastric cancer compared with 2D axial CT: focusing on interobserver variation. *AJR Am J Roentgenol*, 2007,189(2):299–305.

[8] Chen F, Ni YC, Zheng KE, Ju SH, Sun J, Ou XL, Zhang H & Marchal G. Spiral CT in gastric carcinoma: comparison with barium study, fiberoptic gastroscopy and histopathology. *World J Gastroenterol*, 2003,9(7):1404–1408.

[9] Kim JH, Eun HW, Hong SS & Auh YH. Early gastric cancer: virtual gastroscopy. *Abdom Imaging*, 2006,31(5):507–513.

[10] Cidon E & Cuenca I. Gastric adenocarcinoma: is computed tomography useful in preoperative staging? *Clin Med Oncol*, 2009,3:91–97.

[11] Chen CY, Wu DC, Kuo YT, Lee CH, Jaw TS, Kang WY & Hsu JS. MDCT for differentiation of category T1 and T2 malignant lesions from benign gastric ulcers. *AJR Am J Roentgenol*, 2008,190(6):1505–1511.